God has raised up this *Prophetic* and *Powerful* voice to bring healing to many people. I declare that *The Healing Chamber* will be a source of light in the innermost being of the soul, body and spirit of mankind. May it be as *living words*, that move across waters to recover those who need to be healed. I prophesy that the words that proceed from these pages will not return empty, but accomplish healing, as it was purposed to do so. May multitudes *read it repeatedly*, until they are fully healed and whole. It is destined to transform lives.

Prophet Richard D. Sanchez, Servant of God

Everyone is placed in this world for a purpose and will contribute someway, somehow to the human race, good or bad. When I first met Tamonya, it only took me a few days to realize that she was special, and that time will wait for what she can bring. I need not say anything more except to invite the reader to discover Dr. Sands as she unravels herself in *The Healing Chamber*. You got into the chamber, you will come out different from your former self.

Tony Cazeau, MD, JD, Pulmonary/Critical Care Medicine

The Healing Chamber, it gives me great honor to encourage anyone who desires to be set free in their spirit, soul and body to embrace the *life lessons* and many overcoming obstacles and breakthroughs that are taught in this book. As you read this book be prepared for a *renewed mind, transformed body* and a *revived soul*. As I was reminded, I urge you to get ready for the manifestation. 1 Thessalonians 5:23 "And the very God of peace sanctify you wholly; and I pray God your whole spirit and soul and body be preserved blameless onto the coming of our Lord Jesus Christ."

Prophet, Dr. Stephen C. Munroe, Founder, Senior Pastor, Believers Embassy International Nassau, Bahamas

This book is a *declaration* of healing. It is a *transparent, powerful* and *transformative* tool that will literally shift the trajectory of your life. Read it and allow the Master to do His handiwork in your life.

Ursula Chisholm, Vice President, Women Breaking Forth Global Ministries

Tamonya Chisholm-Sands is the daughter of an outstanding Bahamian Christian couple in New Providence Bahamas. I have known this brilliant young Christian lady all of her life from childhood. She graduated from High School and later pursued her Medical Degree abroad. Tamonya continues to be focused, dedicated and persistent in her quest to fulfill her life's purpose. She seeks to deal with healing of the mind, body and soul. My ultimate prayer is that each person who reads ——*The Healing Chamber* — would experience the healing of their mind, body and soul and a greater appreciation of God's love.

Vylma B. Thompson-Curling... J.P., OB.E., M.A. Dip of Ed.

Dr. Tamonya Sands, a true woman of God, who practices, lives and experiences the Word, and it is through this journey, that she has found and experienced God's promise of healing. She shares her own journey to wholeness, by walking with God through diversions, bottlenecks and moments of undesired but purposeful, God ordained stops. *The Healing Chamber* is where you too will experience God's healing touch.

Yvonne S. Bogle, Minister, Women of Worship Ministries, East Longmeadow, MA

Every word that comes out of the mouth of Dr. Tamonya Sands is sanctioned by biblical principles. She is an anointed woman of God with the gift of healing of the mind, body and soul. She can help you bring the broken pieces together, to make a new vessel ready to be used in God's service. I highly recommend this *anointed masterpiece!*

Dr. Sally Taylor, Family Medicine Specialist, Nassau, Bahamas

The Healing Chamber is a *mus*t read, as it provides the reader with meaningful tools to embark upon the healing process as human beings. It allows us to invoke God in our lives to fully receive his healing to be resilient and find our true happiness, purpose and success.

Cranson D. Johnson, Deputy Commissioner Tax and Assessment Westchester N.Y.

The *Healing Chamber* by Tamonya Sands. M.D is a beautiful manual of healing that takes you on a self-journey of sensitization of self, acknowledgement of your pains and hurts without dwelling on them, willingness to be healed and the joy of being healed. She was vulnerable enough for us to learn vulnerability and strong enough for us to be strengthened as we take this awesome journey of *Breaking Forth* with her... she is calling us to come take a walk with JESUS through this beautiful *Healing Chamber* and come out renewed and fortified to live that life of purpose and impact we were created to live.... with this book, you have been handed the keys out of that cell holding you in. *Break Forth* and *Break Free* for Christ calls you forth in Matthew chapter 11 verse 28 "...Come to me all YOU who are weary and heavy burdened, and I will give you rest..." I was blessed, enabled and encouraged to break free and break forth on my journey of *self-discovery* and *purpose*. Do you want a *Break* from all that holds you down? Go read this awesome book. Do you desire *Closure* and *Healing*? You will find it in this book. GOD bless you Dr. Tamonya, for this book that will free many and empower more.

Kate Nnanna-Ibemgbo, John-Maxwell Certified Coach, Author, Nigeria Civil Aviation Lagos-Nigeria

The Healing Chamber

By

Tamonya Sands, M.D.

Copyright

All rights reserved under International Copyright Law. Contents and/or cover may not be reproduced in any form without the expressed written consent of the Publisher and Author.

Unless otherwise indicated, all Scripture quotations are from the Holy Bible, King James Version, New International Version, Scripture quotations marked "NIV" are taken from HOLY BIBLE, NEW INTERNATIONAL VERSION. Copyright 1973, 1978, 1984 by International Bible Society. Used by permission of Zondervan Publishing House. King James Version. (KJV), KING JAMES VERSION (KJV): KING JAMES VERSION, public domain..

The Healing Chamber
ISBN: 9798552406647
Copyright 2020-2021 by **Tamonya Sands, M.D**.
Women Breaking Forth Global Ministries
Visit our website! www.tamonyasands.com

DEDICATION

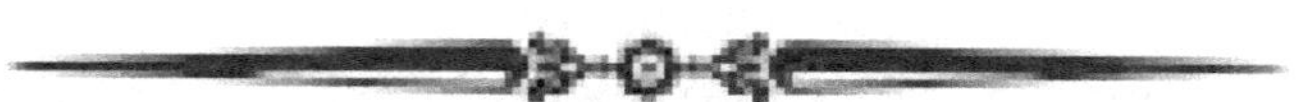

I dedicate this book to my Heavenly Father whose breath gave me hope to live Healed and be made Whole. You have allowed me to walk through much yet emerge refined and unscathed. You were preparing me for this moment. I am grateful for the comfort and direction of the Holy Spirit to pen this book, for the countless souls that have been broken, bitter and pained. You are worth this writing.

I also dedicate this book to my parents Lawrence and Ursula Chisholm who prepared me with a God-centered, integral foundation to provide me with an advantaged starting point in life. I honor you, for every incorruptible deposit, and unbroken love in my life.

Finally, but certainly not trivially I dedicate this book to my husband Thomas whom I love passionately. Thank you for your compassion, encouragement and love. To my Princess Ashera you are my Blessed, Adorable, Fortunate and Favored child. I am honored to have been chosen to mentor you, in the fear and admonition of the Lord. May I be the virtuous model that God purposed me to be in your life. You are both catalysts for my *healing*!

The Healing Chamber!

WHY I WROTE THIS BOOK

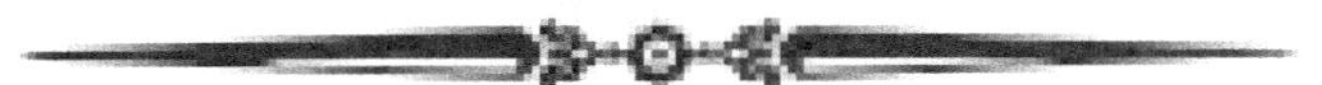

There are multitudes of people traversing the earth, who are broken and need *healing!* It is my supplication that God would use this book to unveil to you His *healing* virtue in your life.

People think of wellness as primarily *physical*, but there are layers of *emotional, mental, financial, social, behavioral, generational, sexual, environmental* and *spiritual* well-being that must come into divine homeostasis for a human to live healed and whole.

You may have been in your condition of brokenness, hurt and interruption for many seasons, but you are about to encounter *"The Healing Chamber"*, where the *Master Healer Himself*, will heal you from the innermost to the outermost layers of your being.

You who are broken, take to the Potter's Wheel and let the process of healing set in motion. This will be one of the most powerful procedures that you ever elected to undergo. Experience the Potter's touch because He wants to put you back together again!

As you turn the pages, may you regenerate, be revived and experience the healing touch. May you begin to *be Enriched, Equipped, Empowered,*

Uplifted and Activated afresh! I pray that by me telling my story, your story will change for His glory! I hope and pray that this book ignites a *chain reaction of Healing.*

"For I will restore health unto thee, and I will heal thee of thy wounds, saith the LORD; because they called thee an Outcast, saying, This is Zion, whom no man seeketh after."

Jeremiah 30:17

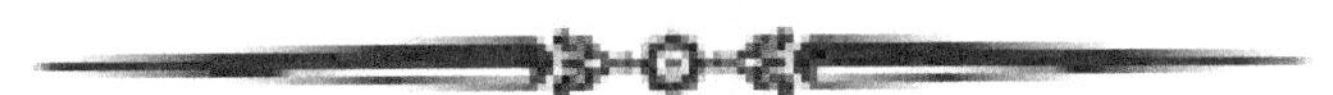

TABLE OF CONTENTS

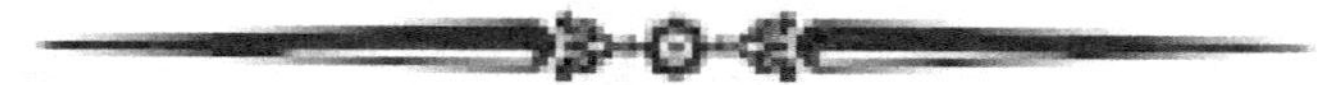

*"I will not cause pain without allowing something new to be born, says the Lord. If I cause you the pain,
I will not stop you from giving birth to your new nation," says your God."*

Isaiah 66:9

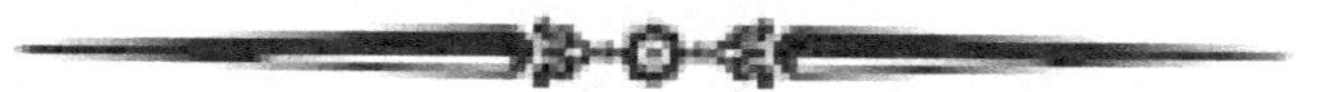

Chapter 1

THE EXPRESSION AND ESSENCE OF HEALING

(The S.G.H of healing)

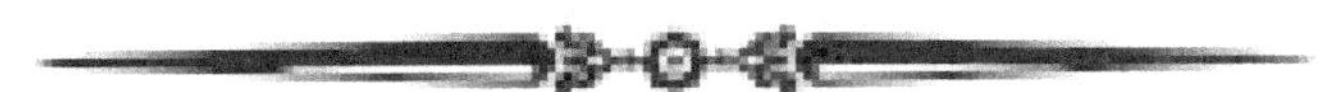

Healing is a gift, a precious gift that everyone including you deserve. God is ultimately the one that bestows healing. "I am the Lord, who heals you." (Exodus 15:26). Healing is a gift that you can procure, but greater it is a gift that you are entitled to. You can secure it and preserve it, through the **S.G.H** of healing.

Healed people know:

- Not to hurt other people
- How to heal other people
- Exist in a healed place

Every utterance, expression and step of your life, should breathe passion and intentionality. The penning down of this book is for those that have been handicapped and bound by strongholds that have been personally, emotionally, professionally, generationally and otherwise linked to your life. These powers have interfered with your ability to breathe and live healed, beyond its expiration date.

It is time to get out of those shackles of the mind, body and soul, but you cannot do it alone.

You have got to partner with a manufacturer or a knowledgeable repairman to repair an appliance under warranty or out of warranty. GOD is the ultimate manufacturer and the trusted repairman through HIS son JESUS CHRIST.

God is the one who heals, He is your ultimate healer. His word was sent to unfasten your shackles, to examine your wounds, and bandage you up.

In order to be healed and made whole, it requires a life transforming decision, that announces that you refuse to remain damaged, partially healed, unsettled and broken anymore. Your being, your existence requires you to declare that you will not live in that state one millisecond longer. You don't need the permission of a perpetrator, parents, best friend or mentor, to move toward a place of healed and whole. Now is the acceptable time for you to propel toward your complete healing, that of the mind, body and spirit!

The childhood hurts, the teenage hiccups, the young adult mistakes are no longer welcome to impede your process. How long will you cling to that which holds you captive? There is no more time for deep-rooted, tormenting pain.

You have borne and lugged your upset, weakness, unforgiveness and damaged soul too long while other people live healed, healthy, successful, whole and full of grace and peace. This moment, as you read this book, is your moment. It is your turn! God has found you and placed this writing in your hands. You must accept and own this gift of restoration to access the limitless life changing opportunities that will be coming your way henceforth.

You have discovered the book that will favor and prayerfully change the trajectory of your life. I have encountered pain and been at a place where I needed healing and to regain wholeness. Now I pray that you can experience the same using the **S.G.H** formula.

S – See the opening for healing and restoration, through the spirit of discernment and wisdom.

G – Glean and be receptive and malleable to the process of healing GOD and those He will put in your path will bring.

H – Have and own your healing. What you own is what you cherish and preserve. Your healing is your right and must be respected by you and all in your life.

"To everything there is a season, and a time to every purpose under heaven." These were the poignant, prudent and wise words of King Solomon in the book of Ecclesiastes 3. Today, choose that it is your time to be healed, and whole. His words are true, but do you believe it? Everything has an end. Let today birth the beginning of a new season in your life.

May the chains that had you bound, release and free you. It is your moment in time to be healed! Declare it, allow it to reverberate in the atmosphere and penetrate your soul. *"This is my moment to be healed."* How many bounteous moments, days, weeks and months are you prepared to exist broken rather than live healed and whole? Do not allow family, friends or co-workers to witness another moment of you being "just okay."

Everything in life that caused you pain, weeping, failures and setbacks did not feel good, nor was it palatable. As a matter of fact, who enjoys being shattered? Nobody! This road called life will not always be fair, the darts will be razor-sharp, pointed and categorically uninvited.

You don't need to accept your hurt and neglect your worry, nor welcome being upset and weak any longer. It does not have to remain a part of your life. You need not be conformed to your pain but declare that you will start to exist transformed because you choose to renew your mind and prove to yourself and others that healing is possible. Do not remain fastened to your discomfort, grief, agony and distress.

Your posture, speech and daily disposition no longer need to emit that you are in a season of brokenness and instability. Your life is about to change, because your mindset is going to shift. You will realize that you deserve more than the irritation but transition into healing. I know that you are wondering how, because you have become accustomed to sitting in that state longer than you care to recall. Declare that this is your Kairos moment, the one that is defining. It's your decisive moment, the one when you consciously decide that this is your turning point.

How can you realize healing and wholeness while being in a state of ruin which limits and blocks your ability to obtain, own and occupy what God has purposed for you? The word of the Lord came to Jeremiah, in Jeremiah Chapter 1:5, "Before I formed thee in the belly I knew thee; and before thou camest forth out of the womb I sanctified thee, and I ordained thee a Prophet unto the nations." God always had plans to prosper you, to cause you to walk in health and wellness. It is now your pursuit, to align your view with God's thoughts, concerning you.

"Beloved, I wish above all things that thou mayest prosper and be in good health, even as thy soul prospereth."

3 John 1:2

Chapter 2

THE OPEN CHAMBER OF HEALING

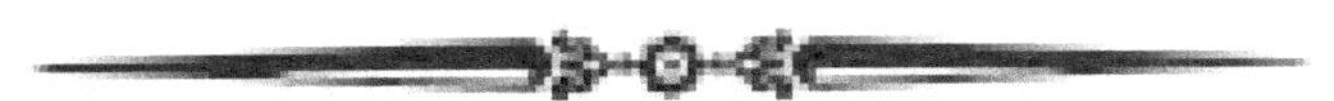

A person can decide to awaken from brokenness and become healed and whole. Healing is not a mystery, it is a posture and a presence. Healing is a daily pursuit. What are you doing every day of your life, to remain healthy, healed and whole? What you do, where you go and who you commune with, can propel you towards a life of healing or divert you from it. You deserve healing! You must decide daily, when you wake up, to pursue healing like you pursue happiness. As a matter of fact, your healing is connected to your happiness.

Here are reasons that you deserve to be Healed:

1. Your faith has been uncovered and magnified.

Blink an eye and realize that God desires you to be healed. When you increase your faith and recognize that you deserve it, you begin to break out of the shell that held you captive and emerge into a place of wholeness. Envision that your faith can move mountains, then you will refuse to remain in the state of trauma and yearn to exist in a space of peace and tranquility.

2. You are willing to conceptualize that you are worthy to walk in healing.

You don't need anyone's recommendation or endorsement to be healed. When you come into relationship with God and you grow in the grace, faith and wisdom of God, you realize that your connection to God, qualifies and entitles you as worthy to walk in healing.

3. Surround yourself with the people necessary to walk healed.

Everyone does not qualify to be a part of your life. Too often people constrict your airway and minimize your oxygen. They compromise your capacity to exist in a space of refreshing, invigoration and wholeness. Identify who is beneficial to your well-being and hold them dear. Minimize or cut off access to your life from those who suck the life out of you. Only you know what you need and can remember what or who lugged you into that painful space not many days before.

The people that contributed to your not too good yesterday, should be put in a place where they can no longer interfere with your well-being. Identify and grant access to the people who have been purposed to advance, propel, and position you for your future, to exchange places with those liabilities of yesterday.

4. Establish a regimen towards daily healing and wholeness

Set out daily to ensure that you walk in a place of healing and wholeness. It is no different from having been ensnared by an addiction to food, sex, drugs or alcohol. You must daily strive to exist in a healed place. Make it your life's work! Pursue it! Your healing is determined by what you do and what you continue to do.

5. Admit that you need God

Your first goal must be a desire to be healed. If you don't desire it, you most likely will not walk in it. You cannot walk in healing without the handiwork of God. With God, your healing is possible. The joy of receiving healing from Jehovah Rapha is that when He does a thing it is well done. He is not like any friend, co-worker, family or associate.

Whatever God bestows upon you, He will never take it back, nor will He remind you of the encounter. "Beloved, I wish above all things that you mayest prosper and be in health, even as thy soul prospereth." (3 John 1:2)

God desires you to live on this earth in a complete state, perfect in mind, body and spirit. Your destiny and purpose are tied up in your healing. You must strive toward His plans for you which are to prosper you and bring you to an expected end. Do you have an expectation of complete healing? You ought to have an expectation! God has a desire for you to be healed. If you knew how to heal yourself, you would have walked in it a long time ago. God is the Master healer! It is time for you to exist in homeostasis, mended, regenerated, revived and in harmony.

While God is the Master Healer, He has gifted someone on earth with whom you can break your silence and divulge your pain. You must emerge from behind the *"pride of pain"* and decide that you will seek out the person who holds your destiny in their hands. No longer can you surround yourself with people who have become comfortable with your unhealed state. Seek and you shall find the person or people that God has divinely assigned to help you work out your deliverance and discover what it truly means to be healed. If your healing is valuable and matters to you, then choose from this moment that it is beyond your time to be healed.

"Therefore confess your sins to each other and pray for each other so that you may be healed. The prayer of a righteous person is powerful and effective."

James 5:16

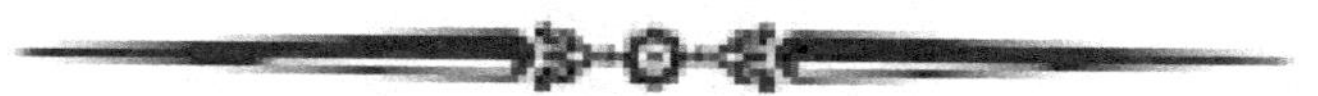

Chapter 3

UNMASKING THE PROCESS OF HEALING

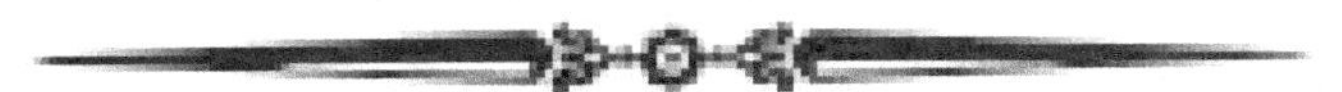

Walking in healing consistently requires you to institute a daily formula, pattern and habits toward your continuous, steadfast healing. Healing is not something you overcome by simply desiring to be healed. Legitimate wholeness in a person's life requires one to visit a moment, a space, a period that they would rather not go to. You must be willing to go to the mournful, joyless, gloomy place, the root, so that you can move toward your desired healing.

Do not continue to mask the pain. Dare not turn your face into a daily routine of work, shopping and baseless schedules because you prefer not to visit the bruised and crushed place. When you wake up every day, commit to engaging in habits and practices that will ensure that your healing is secure. Your purpose is not to persistently return to the harsh truth of what caused you to be in that place, in the first instance.

Every human has the option to decide to do things the same way, with the same people, or to amend their habits so that their future is purposeful and whole. Let the sore habit of being broken go, release it once and for all. It is liberating to begin to ponder and fix your attention on what complete healing could resemble. Believe that you deserve to live healed and whole, but in the power and name of God, not self. Your state of brokenness may have been inflicted by someone, but prohibit them to continue, to have control over your well-being. Healing is a choice that you can create. Make it your new reality. Do things that pursue healing and wholeness. Embark upon a routine that enlists a mentor who can impart tools that can help you.

One day, I decided after many years of dealing with a mother-in-law and her insecurities and Oedipal relationship with her son, my covenant partner, her inappropriateness was not going to sap me one second longer. The days of menace, the moments of invalidation were going to be subdued, by the power of God on the inside of me. I made that decision once and for all, that I would not be a victim and punching bag for her deep-rooted insecurity and disorder. I had developed a habit of resentment but no more, I exclaimed! I had perfected portraying "all was well", to protect *"my business"*, while dealing with "nerve-deep" pain. I sought *"wisdom"* from ecclesiastics, as I preferred wise, biblical counsel.

I disclosed raw detail as the thorns were piercing my flesh and soul. One day, I had a *lightbulb* moment, where I recognized that I needed to change the pattern. My mindset changed! I fortified in God and my strategy for fighting changed. I shifted carnal attire for the whole armor of God. Now, I was ready to battle, in the realm of the spirit against the principalities and workers of darkness at all levels. We all need people, but there comes a point in time when we must do away with running to people for help, and instead cry out to God for deliverance, so that healing could become your bread.

Many people are broken, and they don't even understand the layers of their brokenness. Countless people have adapted to placing bandages on deep wounds, that are infected, gangrenous and will not heal, until they identify and treat the bloodless area, at long last. Past hurt, anger and depression are controlling the daily life of people. Immeasurable pain had consumed my life! I was unfamiliar with such pain and family related disorder, certainly anything resembling this dimension and magnitude. It was an unfamiliar place! Be careful when you marry into a unit or move with a certain group, because you may become a likely target of other people's dysfunction and deep-rooted issues. If you are not prepared, you will adopt it as your own, when it has absolutely nothing to do with you. Realistically, the issue was present before you graced the scene.

The joy of being raised in a family with two loving parents who operated in order and according to the ways of God, was somehow unrecognizable at this juncture of my life. My inherent picture of structure and an outpouring of love and affection was now presenting to me as a demonic Oedipal complex of which I only read about or watched on television.

This new normal was not my cup of tea. I did not like any flavor that was being poured out. As a matter of fact, my preference was no longer tea. The very steam from that cup of tea was repulsive. Either I could allow it to inflame me, as it did longer than required or break free so that I could reclaim my peace, sanity and creativity once again. I had to remember that I entered this space a smart, accomplished, creative woman who had sacrificed years of her life, to become a medical doctor. I had to redeem what the enemy had stolen from me. The cascading series of events had to stop in my life. I had to come to a place where I remembered that God had a mold for me to fit in, which was being blinded by the wounds of what I was experiencing.

Many times, we must take this journey back into who we were before we became who we are now, to know where the cord got broken. We must retrace our steps to the Master Potter so we can fill up those cracks and be whole again.

Brokenness is deceptive! It will take a healthy, successful person and turn them into an addict of pain, suffering, shame and neediness. This kind of person disinherits purpose and the insurmountable time that they invested in achievement. If you don't grab a hold of the situation, time will vanish like the wind, while the mask of the pain consumes you. Be willing to take off the mask, quit pretending and making people believe that you are well. Commit to doing the necessary work to heal. You must be healed. It is non-negotiable! I have come to realize that you have no business, if it is business that is eating you alive while pain consumes you. In other words, how is *"your business"* working for you, by keeping it to yourself, while you die a slow death?

Bitterness and rejected energy must be released. Tell the truth about the choices in your life that may have landed you in the present predicament, so that you can release the torment, become undamaged and release buried, fathomless pain. Developing a habit of walking in freedom and healing must become a lifestyle. Healing has a presence! Its aura is stimulating, revitalizing, rejuvenating and revivifying.

Rotating thoughts of what you endured are immobilizing. It will literally anesthetize you from the reality of freedom and peace. Do not allow your mind to be consumed by it. What you allow to fuel you, will consume you. "Do not conform to the pattern of this world but be transformed by the renewing of your mind. Then you will be able to test and approve what God's will is—His good, pleasing and perfect will." (Romans 12:2).

Daily discourse about your situation will consume your life. God desires you to be free and your heart to be full of joy. Do not allow your mouth to continually give power to your hurt without the purpose of being toward healing and wholeness. In other words, do not speak simply to share the pain, but speak to be freed from the pain.

Choose wisely who you speak to! If they are not helping you, they are hurting and feeding your incompleteness. Today, decide that you will not allow pain to have words anymore, to thrive and flourish, and be glorified in your life. It is time to embrace and clench your healing.

Declare it!

Pursue it!

Just embrace it!

In order to walk favorably, and happily, in the path of restoration there must be:

- Deserving and virtuous reflection and meditation

- God breathed words and conversation
- A plan and vision for your life and your future
- A pattern that is revolving and renewing
- Worthwhile pursuit of what fuels and not breaks you

Choose to magnify and give Glory to the God who can solve your problem, rather than the problem itself. Many people, including family and friends conspire to give energy to your pain and hurt. They feed from your fruitless, failing life. You must pause and ask yourself the hard question of who in your life has the anointing to birth and coach you into healing and wholeness? Who is that person or are the people in life, known or unknown to you, but no secret to God, that walk-in fruitfulness that you can learn and osmose from? Discover who lives a purposeful and successful life and glean from them. The Bible is inundated with scriptures of healing and wholeness. When you are in the company of positive people, your demeanor and spirit should automatically shift. Adorn yourself daily with the word of God, declare and decree His word daily over your life. That is what forward-looking, productive, affirmative people should bring to your life. Everything that you need is in the Constitution of the Word of God called the Bible.

Open it!

Uncover it!

Use it and grow from it!

I have often heard people echo that when they spoke to specific individuals something in their life shifted. Your words, your hope should transmit to others. The doom or gloom, the blessing or wholeness of a person should be reflected in your life, if you spend time with them. Everywhere you go, you should be able to sow seeds of life into people. Someone else should be able to water it, and God will do the increase of what was planted. God desires you to be healthy, healed and whole. This is Gods idea of success in the life of His creation. It is time to recognize who you are in God. It is time for you to discover and walk in your daily healing. Invest your energy, time and resources in discovering the obsession toward healing and wholeness in your life.

"Heal me, LORD, and I will be healed; save me & I will be saved, for you are the one I praise."

Jeremiah 17:14

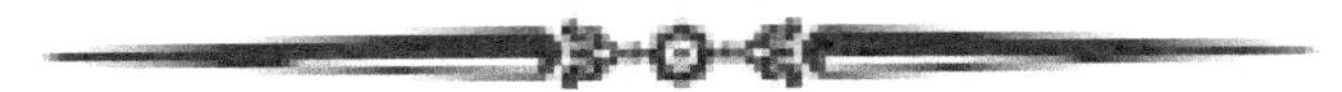

Chapter 4

THE RAW TRUTH & PRINCINPLES FOR HEALING

The spirit of abandonment has been a major contributor to the dysfunction in people's lives. Mounted pain and advocating for everyone else and not self, is commonplace. Many people have and continue to compromise their peace and happiness for other people. It is called sabotaging inner peace and healing for every human while you remain shattered and in pieces.

Be intentional!

Fight for you!

Refuse to be abused and misused one second longer!

When you decide to turn back to God, the person who has the authority and Omnipotence to heal you, then your freedom to live shall be restored. You can be healed! Oftentimes people inherit a state of trauma in their lives, other times, it is self-inflicted. You must be willing to face the truth and differentiate from inherited and self-inflicted wounds. Healing is necessary for the inherited and self-inflicted trauma, but until you can face the gut-wrenching truth, that you did not deserve what was handed to you, and move beyond blame, you will not be able to heal.

Take responsibility for the self-inflicted wounds. Address it! Allow God to heal you completely! A life of prayer will initiate and activate your healing. Open your mouth and begin to cry out to the God of Abraham, Isaac and Jacob. Cry aloud and don't hold back until you receive your healing.

Routine of a person who is fully Healed

1. **Stretch in the morning believing that you are Healed**

   You should no longer be concerned about the struggles and pain of the past, when you wake up every morning. Your focus needs to be on the mercy of a brand-new day and the expectation and assurance that God accompanies you wherever you go. Magnify your confidence! Posture on Faith boulevard! The Prophet Jeremiah wrote in the book of Lamentations "Great is His faithfulness; His mercies begin afresh each morning." Let that mercy give you wings to soar.

2. Never launch your day without consulting God

Imagine daily showering and getting dressed to go to work. When you arrive to initiate your day, there is an exuberant exchange expressing good morning to your colleagues and bosses, mind you the God who blessed you with healing and wholeness has not heard or received gratitude hours into your daily routine. Your daily routine should begin with adoration, praise and thanksgiving to God the second you open your eyes and realize that His breath still perfuses your lungs. There are places where God speaks audibly and transparently. Discover that place where He meets you, just you and Him, and make it your altar. You can term that place, **"Your Healing Chamber"** because it is the place where you encounter God and always experience His healing virtue. It can be anywhere, just make sure that you have that intimate time with Him before meeting others. It brings about clarity, direction, confidence and positivity.

3. Maximize your dependence on God

Healing is fully dependent on trusting in God. It requires the direction, intelligence, power and wisdom of God for complete healing. The guidance and support of friends, family, coaches, even a Pastor is notable, but ultimately you need God. Referring to another human has its pros, but do you really know and understand the characteristics and attributes of the person you are depending on? Devote time to learning and understanding who God is. Open His word and uncover the secrets of Jehovah Rapha, your healer! God sent His word to heal mankind, including you, so uncover the healing power of God through His word. Hide His word in your heart so that it sustains you. What you swallow is what infuses your being and governs your thought process. Plant inside of you what you desire to exist in you!

Bona-fide healing!

4. Clothe yourself in the right garments

Don't let anyone fool you! People who are depressed retreat to dark rooms, and remain in unchanged clothing for hours, even days. Their attire is identifying with a spirit. When you wake in the morning be resolute and purposeful about what you clothe yourself in.

What you wear is a declaration of how you feel. Declare healing and wholeness by your silent, but audible attire. The wardrobe of a person who is abused, hurt, bitter or hurting oozes of barren, tattered and torn apparels. Clothes have an incredible ability to infuse and boost your healing. Do not conceal your pain with clothes but put on garments that boost your spirit and propel you in a favorable direction.

5. Rest assured that God orders your steps daily

This is the time for you to grasp that you deserve to live daily *with* purpose, and *in* purpose. Establish as your *modus operandi* that you will only speak words of power, triumph and restoration. As you invest in every other aspect of your life, you must invest even more into your soundness, stability and completeness. You have been given the key, go ahead and walk out of that jailhouse of pain, insecurity, fear, despondency, faithlessness and dejection into the sunshine of overall wholesomeness.

"'Nevertheless, I will bring health and healing to it; I will heal my people and will let them enjoy abundant peace and security."

Jeremiah 33:6

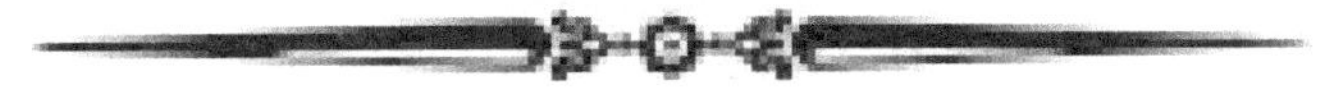

Chapter 5

PURPOSEFUL AND INTENTIONAL HEALING

Dwelling in a broken place drains, exhausts and depletes your thoughts and ability to devote attention to what is purposeful and intentional. I had to make a willful decision that what bankrupted me last season, will no longer have a place in my life, this season. My energy is now strategically devoted to creating a life inundated with people and things that will contribute to my wholeness. Be purposeful, not to revisit the places, where pain and brokenness engrossed and choked your resourcefulness, vision and genius. God placed in you an ability to be an artist, to invent, inspire and accomplish a plethora of things, do not throw your brush away into the trash.

Never allow circumstances or people to have the power to set you back, and impede the blueprint that God designed for your life. The word of the Lord came to Jeremiah declaring his appointment before he ever graced the earth. He was stamped to become a Prophet to the nations by God. Recognize that humanity cannot determine who you will become. All you need to do, is follow the pattern of God, and you will walk deliberately into the plans that He has for you. Either you will believe or not believe the Word of God, the truth is that HE has a divine and beautiful purpose for you, find it, accept it, embrace it and live it!

The plan is already outlined and set for you, to live healed and to succeed. You have been purposed to pursue God, who has the master plan, for your life. As the person desiring wholeness, begin to seek God. Allow Him to begin the redemptive work and unchain the shackles, so that you may experience His presence. Commit to letting go of the things that interrupted your airway for countless minutes, hours, days and years. There must come a point in life, where the chirping of birds makes you smile, the echo of voices excites you and the crashing sound of waves refreshes your spirit and soothes your soul.

A significant part of the healing process begins with implementing an intentional map. A map to follow, so that you are aware and clear of the path forward. An alcoholic needs an accountability system that is reflective of one that a broken person needs to become and maintain healing. This may require a coach, or many coaches. A Pastor or Minister can be an effective resource favoring healing. Discover them! They are to be a source of power, substance, support and inspiration for you.

With the same routine that one wakes up and decides to eat, shower and pursue their day, is the same consideration one must think towards their peace and tranquility. It requires a vow and promise to oneself! Do not allow yourself to set foot in a space of wavering and feeble-mindedness. Prevent your thoughts and emotions from being tested again, because of unpreparedness and not committing to doing the work. Disrupt the pattern permanently! Take hold of that blueprint and move!

There are many places in the bible where God disclosed a plan. Solomon was given the plan for a beautiful Temple. Moses was instructed on the layout and plan of the tabernacle. If God could download to those men blueprints and fine details to curtains, a candlestick, the covering, length, height and sacred cubits then surely, He is well able to reveal the plan that you require to maintain a healthy and structured life. Burst forth, and proclaim, that purpose cannot be fulfilled without a plan.

Organize your days as deposits to organizing your life

1. When your life is organized and prepared in anticipation, it secures you, and ensures that you devote dedicated time and energy to people and things, that will benefit and advance you. Do not connect with people who will assume you as a suitable host, while

stripping you of all of the nutrition that you need to maintain homeostasis of your personal body, mind and soul.

2. You cannot be all things to all people. You cannot climb and ascend ten mountains simultaneously and unaware. Commit to centralizing your thoughts, and zooming in, on what inspires and will propel your life. You can never pour from an empty cup. Fill up before pouring out!

3. Once you transition from broken to healed, your womb speaks to you. You know the feeling of nausea so your guard is erect to repel anything and everyone that will cause you to regress. Organize your life so that you can regain lost moments, hours, days, weeks, months and years. Now, accelerate into realizing your dreams, and embracing your purpose.

When dawn breaks, and you emerge from your bed, ensure that you have more than an idea, of what you hope to accomplish for that day. If you fail to set a plan for your life, someone else will. People always have things for you to do, which has nothing to do with you or your purpose. Daily, set out to reach the mark. Unhealthy pursuits will create unhealthy connections. When your life is organized, and your accomplishments numerous, every facet of your life will be ordered. Ensure that in every sphere of your life you make it crystal clear what is allowed, and what is disallowed in your life. This will maintain a healthy and peaceable space, for you to exist in. Create boundaries!

I have always considered myself one to have a sound foundation on which to compose and establish my life. I was blessed with exemplary guardianship and a wealth of wise examples of what success resembles. I theorized that I had prepared well, in order to face life's hiccups and patiently maneuver the bottlenecks of life. I also believed that some people that were graciously a part of my life intimately or distantly, or by association, were to be vessels that God would use, to inspire and mentor me additionally into my destiny. Their obedience or failure is to be reviewed.

Be mindful of people who welcome your company, but deposit minimally if any, to your being a part of their life. Oftentimes you will come to recognize that your company benefits them, rather than you genuinely being a welcomed guest that they want around them. They use your presence to smooch off your wisdom, spiritual strength and guidance, all the while bankrupting you and you don't even realize it. They deposit just enough to benefit themselves but withhold the cardinal pieces that they can contribute to your development and advancement. It is a well-crafted seduction plan, intended to deprive you. You hemorrhage, almost exsanguinate to death! I understand being left in a fissure without life saving measures. The Supreme God of Supernatural makeup, preserved me, so that I did not lose my spirit and soul and cease to exist.

My creativity was zapped! I couldn't seem to advance! I had prepared to attain what I deemed success, but it was creeping, not happening at the pace and in the manner that I expected. The very thing that I purposed to accomplish, the years of arduous work and commitment was not manifesting the way I had envisioned. I was beyond human repair, but not Jehovah Rapha's restoration and recovery. Seek God on location! It is a topic of its own but plays a major part in prosperity in one's life! Ask Abraham, the Father of Many Nations who was called by God to leave his own country and people and go to a land which was unheard of. His obedience and change in location made him the founder of a new nation.

It was my greatest bitter cup! I empathize with your bitter cup! Mentoring is a biblical principal. My expectation was not far reaching. Moses mentored Joshua, Eli mentored Samuel while Mordecai mentored Esther and Naomi mentored Ruth. Finally, and profoundly Jesus mentored twelve disciples and then He released them to go and reproduce what He placed inside of them. People desire and need mentors to push them and even midwives to birth them into their destiny and purpose. Eager *mentees* show up, ready to learn, but the *mentor* is blindfolded and incapable of fulfilling their role, purposefully at times. This is a deadly connection which could discourage a mentee permanently, if not for the grace of God and mercy of another gifted vessel who has the grace to discern the condition of their soul.

God is a God of grace and He will never fail or abandon you. He will fetch and restore you. One thing I love about God is that He will not leave you comfortless and unprepared. He will send a person who is as qualified, or more qualified than you, carrying everything in them that you need. Be encouraged by this and pray for a discerning spirit to pinpoint them when you meet them eye to eye.

I pray that as I continue to be mentored, in my competence and own leadership, that I would be obedient. I am heartened in my assignment to mentor and midwife those that God has assigned to my life. Somebody's destiny is connected to me. Guess what, somebody's destiny is connected to you too, yes YOU, reading this book. There is a reason why you came across this book, now do not say you are not qualified, HE qualifies whom HE calls and does not call those who are qualified by the standards of the world. You must heal and become who you need to be for those assigned to your life. It is painful when you know that God assigned an individual to help you, but they neglect to do so. That is not your place. If they missed God, they must take that up with Him. Many mentees have already done the foundational work, but simply need the supplementary wisdom from that chosen individual to cross over into the Promised Land. Imagine Canaan being in sight, after you have waded through the barren wilderness, only to have view, but not be able to access it.

The disheartening feeling and moments of gasping for air, but God secured me. I had hidden His word, deep in my heart, enough to preserve me, so that I did not have an unbalanced episode. I never resorted to indulging in spirits, or dependence on any substance to numb the pain. God deposited ample supply of His word in me, over my formative years to nestle me. I knew within my heart that the day would come, when God would shift my life, in the direction that He originally purposed!

Job was tempted by the devil. The prince of darkness could only do to Job, what God had ordained. I have come to realize that God in His Omniscience knows who He could entrust with your life. He already knew who would not fulfil the role, but there was a greater lesson to be learnt by you, for His Glory. People cannot control your destiny, you do! Once you obtain the tools needed to maneuver life, it becomes effortless. You will never realize how much you need healing until you are in an unhealed state. If you are broken, you must enter the Healing Chamber.

The Healing Chamber is not the latest style, it is an *encounter*, a supernatural place, a paradigm shift that is necessary for human transformation. God unveiled it to me, because I had to encounter Him in *The Healing Chamber* so that I could be made whole. I was placed on the wheel, turned, refined, and purified until God processed me to come forth as gold. God had to unmask and strip me! He placed me into the secret, intimate chamber, where I could weep, retreat, lay, rest and recover from the wounds that penetrated my soul. In those moments it became a *Judgment Free Chamber!* While God was working on others, He was supernaturally natured to focus and work on me. I entered the chamber broken but emerged healed and whole. God can do the same for you!

God ministered to me. He can minister to you! Jesus, His Son, encircled and wrapped me in His arms, until every layer of pain exfoliated, and shed from my core. God transfused His whole, redemptive blood into me and saved my life. His procedures do not have adverse reactions. It is all favorable! God summoned me into the chamber, where His outstretched arms embraced me. He did not place me into the hands of man, but He did the intricate work. God the Father, His Son, and the Holy Spirit! Mount the wheel and allow the Master

Sculptor to mold and put you back together step by step exclusively.

The day God spoke and instructed me to be the keeper of *"The Healing Chamber Encounter"*, I knew it was not just another gathering. It would be a chamber, hosted by the King of Kings, where people could enter and be touched by God.

Chambers in the Bible

- Bridal
- Healing
- Gathering
- Guard
- Rest
- Scribe
- Upper

Anyone who authentically encountered God, in the chamber, would never be the same. The time with God would be life changing. I implore you to posture like Daniel! Open your mouth and begin to pray and seek God continuously until He responds, and breakthrough is realized. *He will come*! It may not be when you want Him, but He will surely be on time. Initiate a *Spirit of Gratitude* until God gives you a lasting miracle. The Holy Spirit engaged me in the chamber because I had grasped the rules of how to engage Him. He will meet face to face with you too. Let go and let God minister to you! Be healed and endowed with the Holy Spirit while in the *Healing Chamber*. Partake in the Upper Room experience, while in the *Healing Chamber*, encountering God.

It is my prayer that you will in faith, step into the *Healing Chamber* and allow God to perform Supernatural surgery on you. Let Him do His perfect work, from the crown of your head to the soles of your feet. Trust the Great Surgeon, God! Negotiating with people is one thing but when the Potter wants to put you on the wheel, don't resist it! Surrender and allow Him to put you back together again.

Let God be God!

People may have abandoned you, but God will never leave nor forsake you. He was there all the time, Trust the creator. Begin to praise God. Clap unto Him for the work He is beginning in you. A broken heart impeded your judgement, but do not let it obscure you from the rescue of the Master. The trauma was inflicted, the wounds were great in your mind's eye, but do not allow it to cause you to walk in unforgiveness, forever. When the *Healing Chamber* opens, the fluctuating sweep of human thoughts must surrender to the purging of the Holy Spirit.

I recall being an eager teen in the Bahamas and having the opportunity to work with the Paramedic services on the island, as I knew that I wanted to become a Medical Doctor. An emergency call came in, requesting help for a shipmate who was stranded on a freight ship just off the coast of the island. The man had severed a limb and the ship would not reach land for a few more hours. A strategic plan was implemented where the Chief Paramedic along with one other medical personnel could board a speed boat and venture into the dark, blue, tossed and turning seas to rescue him. I was bold and courageous, and I accompanied the medic without hesitation. I didn't ask the permission of my parents to leave land to sail the ocean for a patient. As far as they knew, I was on land fulfilling my learning experience. God will not hesitate when it comes to His children. When you are bruised, battered and exsanguinating, He doesn't need anyone's permission to leave the *Heavenly Throne Room* to come and attend to you.

Unforgiveness is a virus to your soul! It is compatible to a millstone around your neck, which is an obstacle to your healing. Many people have walked the road that you have. Jesus endured unimaginable pain, betrayal and denial. Let people go, don't begrudge those that you think owed you a mentoring hand. Do you not understand that your life is ultimately in God's hands? Humanity cannot do anything to you, without it being first ordained by God. Your expectation must be directed to God. Shift your destiny, and birth out, what God gave you to produce. Discover resources and people who have been endowed from on high to intercede, push, favor and command doors to open for you.

Everyone will never have an appreciation for your desires, vision and pursuits, quite like you do. God has a perfect plan and desire for you. There were life lessons, that you had to become versed in. God desires people to arrive at a place, where they understand that He is the ultimate source, and mankind is merely a resource on earth. Discern who is an authentic asset to your life. Categorize people according to their role in your life. Ask God to connect you with the people that He has assigned purposefully to your life. Do not live with unforgiveness. Release people, so that you can flourish, thrive and be enriched. You deserve favorable vigor, soundness and healthfulness in your body, mind and soul.

You have lost enough time, being dazed by people who want you to trail them and satisfy their artful deceit, while ensuring that you never align with, or succeed them. It is time to transfer that unfavorable energy from your season of failure, and those who failed you, into a life shifting move.

Mind shift!

Goal shift!

Life shift!

And if he trespass against thee seven times in a day, and seven times in a day turn again to thee, saying, I repent; thou shalt forgive him."

Luke 17:4

Chapter 6

RELEASE PEOPLE, NOT GOD THE HEALER

God doesn't cause people pain, plight, pang, persecution and bankruptcy. It is the Father's good pleasure that you prosper and be in good health even as your soul prospers. Do not confuse the Life Giver with those that caused you pain. I am aware that it is painful to accept that you have missed cardinal moments that you consider permanently lost. Sure, you had some major setbacks! Remember, that a thousand years is but a day to God. God's ways are not man's ways!

God can restore everything that *"went off course"*, that you may have forfeited in life and bring it right back on course as He has the masterplan and the compass of each of our life's journeys. Restoration is a promise from God! For one minute, consider that the road you chose may not have synchronized with what God desired for your life. God had to allow you to go as far as possible down your chosen path, only to teach you a lesson that would benefit you for the path He purposed for you. God is wise and all knowing, He knows when to disconnect dots, while shifting and connecting dots on the predestined path, that He has for you.

Today, as a matter of fact, now, with this gift in your hand, as you stare at this page, this trajectory shifting tool, make the choice to allow faith to bring you back to a place of alignment, order and prosperity. New mercies betide new grace! New grace presents new opportunities! Doors that were prohibited from opening, God will now open. Channels that were delayed are now opening, and things are accelerating and flowing in your direction, so I admonish you in love to MOVE!

The master key to your healing and purpose has always been in the hands of God. Embrace the treasures that are now being opened unto you and placed into your hands. This is an eye-opening moment; it is God who opens doors and God who determines whether a door will remain closed. Only God can touch people's hearts. He desires you to walk in favor with God and man. Things that were once denied will begin to be approved for you. Your failures will begin to turn into successes. The tide that was moving away from you, will shift toward you and eventually launch you in the direction you were purposed to go.

Failure to man is not failure to God. Put it in your grey matter that people do not determine your destiny. Humans are not the measuring stick for your success. Learn it, so that you will be free. Healing is something that if you have it, and you give it away, you will continue to walk in healing and wholeness as soon as you key back into your healing portal. It is always open and ready for you, with God waiting in love.

**"It is good for me that I was afflicted, that I
might learn your statutes."**

Psalm 119:71

Chapter 7

GET UNSTUCK! IT'S A CHAMBER SHIFT

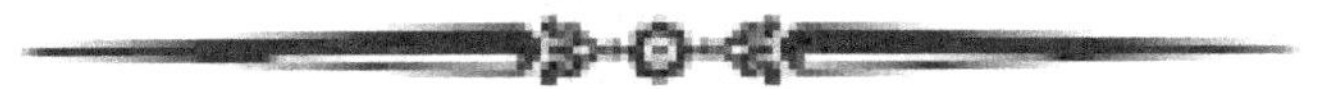

Jehovah Rapha is the ultimate healer. He has the power to heal anyone and everyone, including you. When a person is in a pure relationship with God, they can walk in complete healing. Recognize that everything you endured was working for this season of your life. Understand that your good was considered in it, all along. Once you grasp the healing virtue of God for your life, you will absolutely understand and agree that the pain was for the birthing of a greater purpose.

It had purpose! Satiate and fuel on that!

If you were not afflicted, you would not be able to understand that God could deliver you out of the adversity, the affliction and the peril. You had to be tested, to be proven! It was a faith test! Not every mentee is seeking to be connected to a mentor for monetary gain. Many genuinely honor the mentor and seek their wisdom and leadership to mature in an area that they desire to advance in. Thank God for being tattered, pulled, broken and torn. Now you are ready to shift from stuck to unstuck.

Heal from that place of human disappointment. Hurt is deceptive! When you think that you have conquered it, the thought or mention conjures up emotions that can poison your spirit afresh. You must heal from the seed, not sown by those you hoped would have invested in and guided you. Their missed opportunity need not become your eternal pain. Recognize that the greatness inside of you ignited a spirit of intimidation in them, that they could not give the slip. Pure hearts can celebrate you, but not everyone is mature and gifted enough to take under one's wing and propel others to greatness.

Your feet wobbled transiently, now raise it, and place it ahead of the other. Begin to saunter into your healed place. Let your lift and legacy speak for you, from an elevated, healed place. I reiterate, release it! Listen, let it go! You have come through, to emerge fairer and better than before. You carry a grace and tenacity to withstand thunderstorms, firepits and tumultuous waves. Like gold purified through fire, you must blaze your worth and live it.

Pain can be multileveled and multifaceted. When you dissect the layers, it is crippling. Listen to me my dear friend, allow your setback to set you up for a thrust and rocket into the face of destiny. No season lasts forever, as expressed earlier. This is a brand-new season! When all was said and done, I matured! I had an Epiphany! I wasn't in that necessitous place anymore. The things I desired to satisfy me in practice, self-minimized. I began to truly latch a hold of the scriptures, especially those that admonished me to seek God first, and all other things would be added unto me.

Do you remember King Solomon? God asked him what he desired. The King never asked for wealth, but he prayed for wisdom and knowledge from God. God was so pleased with what was in the heart of Solomon, that He not only granted Him his request, but added riches, wealth and honor. I have learnt to inquire of the Lord with a pure heart and allow God to add the other blessings. Again, people do not control your destiny. God does! You need the influence of God, in your life to be healthy, healed and whole.

When people are hurt, human lens can be clouded as to what people should and should not be doing in their life. Could it be, that you missed the authentic person, who God sent in your life, because you were stuck on the decorated, glamorous looking person? The duplicity of people can have you spellbound and missing God in the carnal moment. It is not uncommon for people to present one way, but lack substance.

May the cataract clear, and scales disappear so that you may see clearly, what favors or opposes you. When you become transparent about your life and what has been destabilizing you, then you can move forward, upward and onward toward the rising sun. Glory awaits you! What was once designed to incapacitate and impair your mental ability, even leave you breathless, may it be used as a launching pad for you.

Being afflicted, hard pressed and in pain does not feel good. If you never experience discomfort you will never learn how to authentically appreciate the precepts of God. The book of Psalms awakens us to a righteous being who encountered trouble after trouble, but God will always bring you safely to shore. Nothing in life that you encountered and weathered, stunned God.

What you were humanly unable to accept and grasp yesterday, God is now able to unfold to you today and use to guide, assist, minister to and encourage others. See, your story had majestic purpose! Life is not deprived of affliction and shortcomings. God has lined the scriptures with practices and steps to back you in overcoming it. Be healed, by the blood of the Lamb and the words of your testimony.

Generational spirits are a major contributor to brokenness in people's lives. So much of human perils were inherited, certainly not all self- inflicted. Imagine children that were born with congenital issues that have remained to this day. They inherited something that they did not ask for or desire, but they must fight through and not succumb to what was designed to consume them.

You may be the offspring that was conceived in an unhealthy relationship. You may have been shortchanged from having and establishing a relationship with your father, which is commonplace and his other children and your siblings. Perceive that sin was the cause of your lifelong pain! You were not responsible for everything that faith dished out in your life. Perhaps you are the descendant, whose father or mother was an addict, maybe because of their own childhood woes or personal pain. There is no one who doesn't have one form of inadequacy or the other in life, either directly or indirectly.

Any human who was unable to maneuver their private inner pain, will surely be incapable of acquiring the proper tools to nurture anyone. Unresolved pain in one generation, infiltrates its way into another generation and souls are chained, shackled and destinies truncated. May you be the vessel that God uses to break the cycle of generational brokenness. I declare the cycle to be broken.

Pain is subjective! Pressure is objective! Each human has a different threshold for pain but when pressure is applied, if that area is sensitive, you will respond in displeasure, no matter what angle you are touched from. The flesh cannot overcome the flesh. You require willpower, a frame of mind and supernatural power to overcome it. In order to truly become unstuck from the sensation and comfort of pain, you must be willing to shift the blame from people. No more blaming people. Clear the obstruction out of your life so that fresh favor can be poured into your life. God can only pour blessings when you are merciful and sparing.

Early 2015, I received a diagnosis that would have swiped many humans off their axis. I was reminded that those who trust in God cannot be crushed. We must trust God, while we are being pulverized. This is how we are molded and shaped into gold that is pure and that God can use. The six-letter word diagnosis that many have sleepless nights about, did not have authority over me. I walked in authority over it through the power of God that was on the inside of me. I am healed and whole, permanently! I *went* through and *came* through, unscathed! The scar that is permanently impressed upon my chest, post three surgeries is my battle scar! It reminds me of the goodness and glory of God but more the pain that Jesus endured when He went to the cross, just for me. He already bore my encounters on His body on the tree, therefore by His stripes I was already healed.

We aren't afforded the freedom of really choosing from the shelf, what we prefer to endure in this life. It was my test to pass, and God prepared me to transcend it, and emerge pure as gold. God knows the way that we take. After He tests us, He shall find us pure. Guess what, every unsought, undesired test, prepared me for the greater test. The mental, emotional and academic test, which I thought was difficult, was what God used to strengthen my faith muscles for the greatest test of my life, facing a diagnosis of skin cancer. I thank God for the dress rehearsals that I already had, which dressed me to walk through the advanced test. I was prepared! Therefore, I leapt over the hurdle with flying colors. Blessed be the name of the Lord.

I have taken a seat in *the Healing Chamber* for emotional, professional, physical, spiritual, pecuniary and in-laws healing. When God takes you into the chamber, He performs complete surgery! Every facet of your life is inspected and palpated so that post-surgery you can harmonize and operate in divine homeostasis. I was the first partaker of the healing operation. I know what joy awaits you! It is time to be triaged. Get anchored in God! God is God! What He ordains to occur, will occur. He knows the outcome of your surgery. It is time for your head to toe, inside to outside, layer by layer healing. God reminded me that my *"sickness"* was not unto death, but for the Glory of God! When your faith is activated, you will recognize a test posing as sickness. God gives breath and He will take it, on His terms. Do not allow what you see in the natural to take you off equilibrium. It is not really what it appears to be. If you are not prepared when the illusion presents, you will miss the truth and reality of what is being portrayed.

Your pain, setback, limitations and failures cannot last forever. This too shall pass! Weeping is but for a while! By morning time, joy shall wipe away the tears. It was all working together for my good and God's glory! My questions were endless. It was my human nature to inquire of God about my condition. I had sacrificed countless years of my life pursuing my desires, traveled across the globe in pursuit of diverse ways of soaring in my field, only to end up in a predicament I loathe. Was it really a deep-water experience or simply a divine interruption? When you don't have the tools to understand supreme moments of life, it will extend beyond the set time, because you were unprepared for the intermission.

Intermissions are purposeful if used wisely. I accepted that His ways are not my ways and His thoughts not my thoughts. God had a greater purpose for me to impact lives through *education, leadership* and *mentorship* under a *Medicine & Ministry Mantle*. I have been blessed with the gift of healing naturally and supernaturally. It is my prayer that you are healed from the expectations of people, maybe the very ones who contributed to your motionlessness.

Do not become stuck, Get unstuck now...

What happens when a brilliant, accomplished person studied to become a lawyer, thinking that the only place a lawyer can work is in a courtroom? If they are clouded, it will put them in an unbalanced place. Imagine a Fortune 500 company being where God desired them to take and operate their gift. When a person knows what God placed on the inside of them, and that they qualify to operate outside the box, they will soar. I finally understand that my purpose was to operate in my gift uniquely from a *learning, leadership, legislative, specialist* and a *consultative* role. I use my roadmap to prepare thousands of medical professionals for the field according to the gift that God placed in me, intentionally as an accomplished Physician. I am blessed to create another generation of leaders in the medical field and caretakers who would have the pulse of God, while tending to the natural and physical needs of humanity. It took me encountering bottlenecks, more obstacles than needed to wholeheartedly grasp my divine purpose, fully! God gifted me with this divine revelation! I sacrificed precious time, and years being stuck! I was stranded and puzzled for longer than I care to remember. I now choose *not* to live stuck in any area of my life, ever again, but enlightened, flourishing, healed and whole.

Many are misguided even in their recognized brilliance. They are shortchanged from that cardinal piece of the puzzle to mount to the next level. All MD's do not work in a Hospital, as all Engineers aren't employed in a manufacturing plant. It is time to stop presenting these minimized boxes for humans to operate in, because if they don't fit in that box, it can throw a human off indefinitely and possibly shatter them. God created people to be distinct and function uniquely. The ways and limitations of man are not of God. Limitation is not a characteristic of God. It behooves you to learn and govern your life by the ways of God. "Now unto him that is able to do exceeding abundantly above all that we ask or think, according to the power that worketh in us." (Ephesians 3:20)

There is beauty and freedom in recognizing that you are positioned precisely where God desires you to be. He had a global plan for me to impact lives from a unique perspective. My fingerprint, superimposed by His Majestic handprint, is carved in the lives of hundreds, if not thousands of lives forever and ever. Do not become stuck! I pray that my God ordained experiences can be an example that God uses to arrest persons who have experienced temporary hiccups. I pray that you are redirected to the original track that God purposed for you to march on. My *Ministry and Medicine Mantle* include mentoring while precluding people, from experiencing the dragging, wearisome seasons that I endured. People must be able to connect to God, by way of His agents in the earth, so that they can heal, transform and regain their power and purpose in the earth. Mentorship is an underrated and misunderstood gift! Scripture is inundated with examples of mentoring. Every patient, that my students touch and care for, have and will forever have my imprint in their lives. The theory, clinical skills, medical laws and ethics, and words of wisdom and the training that I imparted to them, is being experienced and palpated nation and worldwide.

Do not become stuck!

Healing is connected to deliverance which paves the way for restoration. God never promised you that you would live in this world without trouble, but He assures you that He would never leave you alone for Christ admonishes us to rejoice for HE has overcome the world. Rejoice in hope and persevere in tribulation. Discover how to embrace the tools, that are required to maneuver and surpass the roadblocks in life. Parading the earth with impaired vision is a deadly handicap. With the unimpaired ability to see, everything in life begins to uncloud and illuminate. The lens of your heart can accommodate that rebirth, bringing healing into clear view. The book of *Job* reminds us that blessings can emerge through pain and suffering. The book of *Proverbs*, unveils the wisdom of God for daily living and existence. In the book of *Ruth*, we glean that Ruth was mentored by her mother-in-law Naomi, and ultimately experienced a life of redemption, despite the loss that she along with her family suffered. God's peace is healing! When you discover His purpose and plan for your life, empowerment and enrichment will grace your life. All the sacrificial years were not wasted! I now understand that it was necessary for preparing me for this very moment, where I would pen this book.

My life is deliberate! Your life is deliberate!

My time is purposed! Your time is purposed!

Nothing happens by chance; they are all spiritually orchestrated.

The moments of my life are precious and strategic now. I guard what I grant permission to access and penetrate my ear gate and osmose into my spirit. Commit to doing the same. May every moment of your life be inspired by God and function according to the divine order of God. Brokenness is an expression of disorder.

Operate in the order of God!

When you come into the knowledge of healing, be determined never to allow pain to enter your life again. Allow people in your life, that are looking glasses of what you desire your future to look like. Everyone's emergency is not your emergency. The quickest way to retreat to a dark place, is to dabble in things and entertain people that you have not been anointed to handle. Direct your attention to God for divine instructions concerning everyone who desires to occupy a position in your life. What's their purpose? Discover who and what is integral to your life. Some people are on assignment to loot your hope, interfere with your healing, and hold up your peace. Understand your value and only allow those who honor the gift in you, to benefit from your time and deposits. No looters are allowed! Be alert in the spirit!

Learn to hear from and obey instructions from God. Familial people are satisfied with your commonplace condition. Mentorship and leadership are imperative for a broken person to transition into a healed season. God in harmony with the Holy Spirit will lead, guide and direct you into all truth. The Holy Spirit will never mislead you on what relationships are fitting for your wholeness.

Your life and time are valuable!

Your health and wellness are paramount!

When you are healthy and whole, then and only then, can you create and devote time to focus on what pertains to purpose and success in your life, which will translate to the life of others.

"I have been young, and now am old; yet have I not seen the righteous forsaken, nor His seed begging bread."

Psalm 37:25

Chapter 8

GOD HEALS AND TURNS THE TABLE

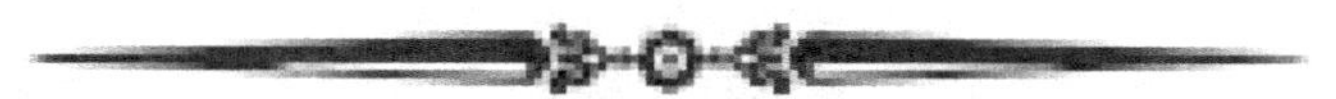

The famous Winans brothers once sang a powerful song called, "Ain't no need in worrying what the night is gonna bring, it'll be all over in the morning." When the rising sun begins to make its appearance over the horizon at daybreak, it signifies the dawn of newness. Morning after morning new compassion, goodwill, grace and gentleness you will see as you embrace healing and restoration. It does not matter the category of hurricane that hit your life yesterday, the sight of sun gracing the earth, signifies and breathes hope. Beaten and defeated you may have felt, but do not permit it to define you for a lifetime.

How long will you allow yourself to be incapacitated by the afflictions of five, fifteen, thirty plus years ago?

How well is that serving you? Use your pain as a lesson and stepping stone to catapult you through the situation, regenerated and rejuvenated. Maneuver from pain to purpose as you birth your gains through your pains.

No season lasts forever! The tables do turn! Winter must cease, so that spring can burst forth. You must say goodbye to summer for harvest to yield! A fractured heart, fragmented spirit and mangled life cannot define you forever. There is an innate voice, a cheering heart that is rooting for you! Hear the voice! Respond to the cheers! Fight and shout loud! Demonstrate that what had you bound, has released you and now you tread upon it. Be healed, completely!

When you arrive at the consciousness that pain and torture has taken its toll long-windedly, and that healing is your portion, it is cathartic and life-changing. Healing can only be secured when you procure the tools and impartation from a spiritual source. Victorious, healed people push and believe that they can break forth unscathed and complete.

God will present you with blessings that exceed what you forfeited. Job received a double portion, twice as much as he lost. Rest assured that it shall come to pass. Restitution shall be sweet! You shall recover it all! Time invested in *Prayer*, *Study of God's Word* and *Worship* will unlock the healing oil of God in your life.

Hurriedly and suddenly, you will be able to stroll into the betrayer, invader and adversary's camp and gather the spoils. Possessions and goods will be at your disposal because you passed the test. Posture yourself before Him and prepare for the greater in comparison to your lost. The worms stole your joy, peace and sanity, but God will make good on what was hopeless. There comes a time when being hurt and vexed and giving power to people and being stranded and perplexed on your present condition must be released.

The suffering that you endured will not be able to compare to the glory that awaits. An awakening of healing puts you on the starting line toward your purpose. Your process toward healing will create growth. Your healing will reestablish vision for your life. Once you are healed, brokenness will be like a putrid fragrance to your existence. Healing will bring you to a point of convergence and prime focus. When you are healed and centered, the spaces and rooms that minimized and underestimated you, will replace with new spaces and new opportunities that will maximize and praise you by God.

I now realize that the anointing that God placed upon my life, came at a cost which took me down the mound, on the backside of the mountain, *in* the pit and *under* the pit. He makes everything beautiful in His time. The *pit* life will shift to the *palace* life for you! When you *suffer* with God, you will eventually *reign* with Him. Favor, blessings, treasures and gifts will be your portion.

When you exist healed and whole, and walk fitly in your purpose, the table will eventually turn. Where you were unwelcomed, you will be invited. Where you were unrecognized you will gain spotlight. You will be requested and desired of mere men. Guess what! What you may classify as the most despised moment in your life, to God, it was only a light affliction. Meditate on that! It was only a light affliction! Your suffering was atom size to God, when you were categorizing it as mega size. The very affliction that you endured will result in a greater glory. "For our light and momentary troubles are achieving for us an eternal glory that far outweighs them all." (2 Corinthians 4:17)

The burning fiery furnace that you survived, will increase the very presence of God in your life. Amid the fire, God showed up and you were not consumed. He will enrich you with virtue and His riches. Fortune and favor, in your life, will be on full display. This read was penned to transition you. The golden moment is upon you. You were in the fire, but today, begins a divine shift in your life.

Think cured!

Think restored!

Questioning God, appears reasonable when you are writhed with pain. It is unimaginable to comprehend that you faced moments in the fire and that you were burnt and received blisters. It is imperative that you move beyond your setbacks! Posture for your comeback! Do not begin presenting numbers and days to God, because it is negligible to Him. Rest in the hope that everything in life has an expiration date!

"But He knows the way that I take; when He has tested me, I will come forth as gold."

Job 23:10

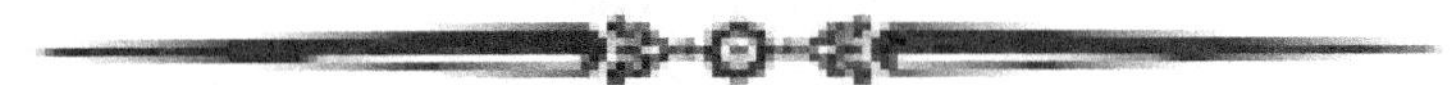

Chapter 9

BREAKFORTH FOR HEALING

Having a flashback on your pit and prison experience is something that is naturally and humanly understandable. The agony, failure and unforgiveness reverberates in your mind, but you must discipline yourself to erase it painstakingly from your mind, except by the words of your testimony. Rise to the occasion of your healing! Challenge yourself to remain on the path of restoration. Engulf yourself with people who uplift and raise your spirit. Reject those who depress and afflict you. Reject anything that mirrors the stinging moments in your life, and the arduous relationships that fought your sanity and peace.

My writing is from a place of authority! I have been there and experienced that! Languished, secluded and disheartened! Recognize when it is time to divorce yourself from the *former season* in your life where you experienced pain and problems. If you don't you will miss what God has for you in *this season*. Refuse to revisit aforetime and shift into your future. The season of discomfort and sadness only prepared you to shift into a season of celebration and manifestation, to partake in every good and perfect gift from God, remember, *old things are passed away and everything has become new....*

Depression has a manifestation that people don't normally recognize. It is called the *attraction syndrome.* Depression is an artful recruiter! Depression knows how to recruit friends, to join the "blue funk and woe" party. Those friends include anger, and the melancholy voice that whispers negativity consistently and persistently in your ear and into your spirit. That sneaky but blatant voice taunts and tantalizes, while enlisting you. The voice creates lies, convincing you that you are enduring your pain alone, and it echoes that nobody seems to recognize or care for you. It renders you cheerless, hopeless, joyless and in an unfortunate stupor. The dismal truth is that you were hair's breadth away from meeting a spiritual, emotional, physical and mental disruption.

The test may have appeared never-ending and as if God never desired to intervene. In the thoughts of Job, would it ever cease? Penning this book is purposeful! My prayer is that my transparency, voicing my *"unhealed season",* will strengthen you, to walk through your season but not to be consumed by it. Once your test ends, you will be able to withstand any weather pattern, any seasonal temperament and hiccup that life presents. I pray that your test will appear accelerated and quickly finish. You know the content now, you understand the questions so hasten, and finish the test. Do not allow yourself to be bamboozled any longer.

It is time to close the book on this chapter of your life!

Complete this chapter, so that you may begin to pen down the new chapter of your life, from a healed, and not a broken place. You have a will to make that decision, at this very moment! You can decide to bunk in the *torture chamber* or make a chamber break and shift into *the Healing Chamber* so that you can be made whole!

Misery is not your portion!

Get a grip on it, now!

Your space of pain, that room that you dwelt and found solace in, it has caught a fire. It has been destroyed and deemed uninhabitable. Make the shift! Replace the pain with purpose! Those giants in your life, have been defeated. Get focused! Procure the tools from God the Father, that you need. Write your script anew! Flip the script on the devil and those who were being used by him to glory in your season of unrest.

Shift your destination and focus on walking fully in your purpose! Redirect your energy, into discovering how to bend the curve! Veer in the direction of strength, progress and freedom. Break forth with favor in your life. You were created to exist healed! I reiterate, pray that God will connect you with a mentor, who will empower, shape, impact and develop you. Your supplication must be to God. It is imperative to study bounteous amounts of the Word of God. Supplementing this with intentionally engaging in activities that you lacked creativity to touch when downcast, would shift the trajectory of your life. Hope thou in God!

All things surrounding God must be your go to! Begin to meditate on scriptures of healing and discover resources that will feed and develop you. The time of pain being hidden in the depths of your soul, have contributed to your interruption and a long-winded coffee break in your life. It stops now! Be intentional about your healing. The benefit of a coach that God has chosen for you can help you to identify and face provocation, ultimately changing the trajectory of your life.

Healing is mental, emotional, physical and spiritual. There must be harmony in all aspects of life, to thrust you in the direction of your divine homeostasis. God created you in order! Choose not to be stuck any longer. The place, things, people and scenes that occupied your life can no longer order and control you. It is misleading to advise you that you can accomplish it cold-turkey! There must be divine intervention, which directs you to natural and human mediation, to interrupt the pattern and shift the paradigm! I pronounce you unrestricted, unfettered and unshackled.

Chains break!

You have now been commissioned, enriched and prepared to launch. Move from the prison of captivity, to the opportunities that have been in expectation of you. Emerge! Overthrow what has been dominating you! Speak to the humps and failures in your life and command them to move! It is time for you to set goals, and create ways to grow mentally, emotionally and spiritually. Your spirit, soul and body must be fed. Shift your gaze upon God first, and then toward things that will cause you to experience the healing power of God. You have done the work, now you can benefit from the work, that you have invested in your healing and hiding place in God.

"But they that wait upon the LORD shall renew their strength; they shall mount up with wings as eagles; they shall run, and not be weary; and they shall walk, and not faint."

Isaiah 40:31

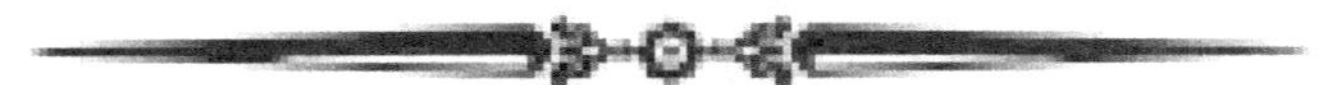

Chapter 10

THE WAITING ROOM

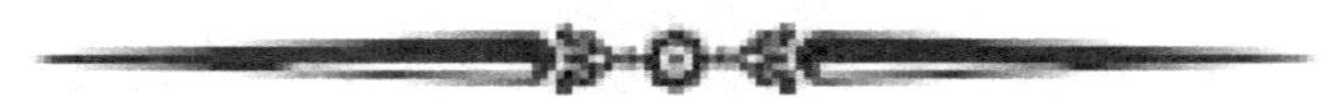

Waiting is an interval! It is a period that requires you to be following instructions, while you are in waiting. It is a test of the essence of your ability to remain poised, patient, persistent and persevering. Jesus already paid the price for your healing. While you wait, wait intentionally and purposely.

Waiting is a:

- Position
- Posture
- Place

How do you wait?

- In Rest
- In Meditation
- In Expectation
- Abiding in Faith
- Focused on the prize

While you are weary and burdened, God bid you to come unto Him and He will give you rest. In God alone, you can find rest. Waiting on anything at all requires patience, while remaining blameless and upright. Waiting patiently does not dismiss the anticipation and expectation to be healed. In truth it requires the one waiting to abide, with a heightened level of faith. Imagine a woman who is with child. When she discovers that she will become a mother, immediately she begins preparation, in anticipation, while waiting for the baby to mature and ultimately be born. Make your waiting purposeful, not wasteful!

Waiting attracts many emotions including irritability, anxiety and even excitement. When you are zoomed in, while waiting and engaged in something valuable, suddenly, in a moment the wait will be over. The sound of a baby crying will greet you. The most beautiful blessing will stare innocently into your eyes. Everything that you endured to prepare for that moment, will be forgotten at the sight of new life!

I will never forget, what was supposed to be one of the most beautiful days of my life, was suddenly interrupted. In an instant, I was facing the greatest challenge of my life. It was at daybreak, *September 12th, 2005* about a week post my expected delivery date, that I began experiencing labor pains. My husband and I pampered our own selves, clutched the hospital bag and journeyed to the hospital.

Upon arrival the midwives got me settled in my room, while I waited for my Obstetrician to check in, on me and the baby. To accelerate labor, he decided to rupture the membranes using a specialized tool. Being that it was my first pregnancy, my husband proceeded to work to clear his desk and return as quickly as possible. As I lay in the bed, anticipating the arrival of our gift (*gender to be revealed*), I was going through the process moment by moment. I experienced labor and delivery many times from the other side of the bed, but I was about to have my own experience as an expecting mother. I called my mother who was across the ocean in the Bahamas, to tell her that I had gone into labor. In that moment the atmosphere shifted. The tempo increased as nurses began to assemble in my room indicating that my baby was decelerating. I was undeterred because I thought the warm fluid flowing from my body was amniotic fluid. I quickly realized that it was more than fluid. Things started to really intensify as well over half a dozen healthcare professionals scurried in my room. With my medical training, but now patient mode, there was no doubt that something major was happening. They attempted to stabilize my baby, by having me shift onto my side to optimize blood flow to the baby.

The urgency intensified as the Physician who was leaving the past nights on call shift, while my Physician stood by, decided to examine me. As he raised the white sheets covering my lower body, we were undoubtedly having a medical emergency, as there was a deluge of bright red blood. I was now the center of a critical emergency. In my immediate distress I managed to remain calm enough to call my husband, as I clenched my cell phone, to gently inform him that danger lurked. My situation was life and death as I was losing more blood than my body could tolerate. I was having a Placental Abruption with massive bleeding.

In the excitement of my *waiting*, I had to shift my focus in a life-threatening moment to calling on the name of Jesus, to heal my child and me, and bring us through healthy, healed and whole. As they bustled me along the halls from the delivery room to the operating room, I started to become weak, and lose my ability to recognize or apprehend what was taking place around me. The room became dim, as I could faintly hear the medical exchange between the nurse who was hoisting me and the Anesthetist, as he attempted to perform an Epidural. The last words I remember interpreting, sounded something like "just get it in." Those words are etched in my memory.

Your faith must never diminish in critical moments of your life. You must be postured to call on the name of God to show up in your situation. Emotionalism will not move God to heal you! Praying and calling on His name will! I had faith to believe that the one who created me and placed a child in my womb, would heal and bring us through. While it was a critical moment, one that I will never forget, there emerged the most precious sound ever, the cry of our baby, seconds after my husband burst through the doors of the Operating Theater in his green scrubs and socks. The Obstetrician was able to place this 6lbs,10 ounces bundle of joy into his hands. Our princess Ashera (*which means blessed, adorable, fortunate, wealthy and ever-increasing strength*) with a head full of silky black hair, peered into my eyes, as my husband held her in front of me, as I lay on the table. Behold what beauty! What the enemy meant for bad, God turned into something precious and splendid. The promise eventually came forth amid going through the valley of the shadow of death. I did not fear any evil, for I knew that God was with me.

Master your waiting room experience! Oh yes, waiting is a gift! Human preference is always for things to happen now especially for those that have endured hardship and been tormented in their spirit. Many invest diddly in the wait, but without incubation, there cannot be manifestation. The woman who had an issue of blood tried numberless ways and duodecimal years to be healed. She was ostracized because of her condition. This gentlewoman wasn't even welcomed to go and worship God. It is unimaginable to consider the countless days that she lived in her undesirable condition. Envision her experience! Explore her perseverance and steadfastness! The woman did not receive her healing at the onset and initially at her desired time. Her faith was tested and magnified over her twelve years of suffering. That is what ultimately got God's attention and eventually healed her! Her faith made her whole!

She made up her mind that she would not live in a hemorrhaged, weakened state one day longer. She refused to live broken anymore. What about you? Are you tired of your condition yet? Can you muster the faith to let go and let God heal you? The enemy has an assignment, which is to glory in your suffering. Today, the peaks and valleys cycles must stop. Refuse to be broken one more day, hour, minute or second. Light upon who you need to locate, so that you can be healed and made whole.

There is One, who holds the key to your healing, and He is called:

- Great Physician
- Healer
- Deliverer
- Jehovah Rapha

Descend upon your creation and make good on your promises Abba Father. Do you know that it is God's will that you blossom, flourish and be in good health? God is the ultimate healer, but He has also graced and anointed someone walking in human flesh to pour into you. It is ever essential that you find that person who can mentor, equip and birth you out of the lifeless place.

Talitha cumi!

Arise, daughter!

Arise son!

Be comforted! Pinpoint and identify the person who holds your breakthrough in their hands. Your season of lavish and perish is spent. Decide this minute that you will unlock delayed promises. Be determined, to discover every hidden treasure, that you are entitled to. Delayed ability to break forth, out of the unrest in your life, is not all self- inflicted. God holds the key to your total life. God allowed you to endure the hardship. If God did not apply the brakes, you may have paraded into danger land. You may have walked into doors that glittered but were not wholesome, for you. Walking into some doors may have carried you into a more devastating place.

Endurance is prescribed, to keep you calm and foster much needed fortitude. The formula was remedied to ensure that you did not interfere with the grand promises and blessings of God for your life. There is a time and season for everything!

Every season of your life is pertinent. When you are capable of appreciating and delighting in the succession of seasons, you will walk fully and wholly in purpose.

A prolonged season of waiting, the season of shaking, turbulence and development was responsible for the birthing of my ministry, called *"Women Breaking Forth."* This ministry was birthed on *May 18th, 2010* during what I would consider the peak of discomfort, in my life. God used the pain, to birth forth purpose! Mentoring and equipping strengthened me and magnified in my life. *Women Breaking Forth!* now breathes to *equip, enrich, educate and empower* people to become who God purposed them to be.

Consider Joseph who had at least ten older brothers and one, who was younger. His brothers were jealous of him, because of their father's deep love for him. Joseph was a dreamer who naively shared his dream with his brothers. He was clueless to the depth of their resentful spirit and disdain for him. They conspired and threw him into a pit. Amid deception and jealousy, God was with Joseph. Joseph endured his test, and God was right there with Him. He never left Joseph alone.

Joseph was subsequently placed in prison for something he was not responsible for. During his captivity, Joseph found favor with the captain of the guard named Potiphar, which resulted in him being put in charge of every prisoner. Joseph's ability to interpret dreams, made room for him, and set him in position to interpret the ruler's dreams. This opened the door for him to run the full affairs of Egypt's ruler. During a time of famine Joseph was put in charge of food. The very brothers, who sold him, had to now come to him to eat and live. God was in the thickness of it all. God never left Joseph. He knew the outcome from the onset. What was designed to cripple you, will be used to bless you. The pit and the prison were *preparation chambers* for Joseph. The *pain chamber* was the *preparation chamber,* to position him to run the *Kings chamber*.

You were overlooked, but now you are in clear view. God has considered, observed and chosen you. Those who did not notice you in old days will be mandated to stand before you in later days, in order to take their next breath. You went through and came through. God will announce your name and bring you into a spacious place. The valley could not contain you, because the palace was calling for you. The very anointing, gift and talent that was hidden, sabotaged and suppressed, God will shift it in favor for your dominance. You are the head and not the tail! You are the first and not the last! You are the chosen and not the rejected of God! You will no longer exist condemned but promoted. Your birthing pangs was a sign that you would come forth stronger, better and healthier than you were before.

The pit of despair, addiction, financial bankruptcy and insufficiency had to release you. It was all temporary! Now, yes now, your permanent space has summoned you. You are no longer confined! Glory comes at a high price. Veritably what was planned for Joseph's detriment, God turned it into his merriment. I declare that you will not breathe your last breath in the pit, but that you shall propagate, bring forth and come forth with a reinvigorated breath.

It is theoretical to dream while in pain, but it also requires one to stretch to emerge redefined. A minor, or major setback, does not define who you are. Everyone must make a pivotal decision. Take the approach of investing in what is necessary to accomplish your goals. Reset and refocus on the things that you initially set out to fulfill. That is ultimately what will define you. Do not allow one human's no, to become your final answer. A yes awaits you, now go discover, recover and uncover it. God is greater, stronger and wiser than anyone and anything. He is healer and possesses the ability to infuse mankind with a vision, and an ability to accomplish it.

Do not waste another moment crying or gasping for air. Behold, the Word of God, the *Constitution* and *Manual* for every life to succeed. Uncover the secrets! Lay hands upon the treasures of God for your life. Pray and seek His face! While you wait, pray! While you wait study God's word! The *waiting chamber* is also a place of renewal and strength so that you can mount up on wings, like an eagle and soar. When it is your appointed time to run, you will not become weary! When you accelerate, you will not faint. There is much to be unveiled while you are in the *waiting chamber*.

"Not only so, but we also glory in our sufferings, because we know that suffering produces perseverance; perseverance, character; and character, hope. And hope does not put us to shame, because God's love has been poured out into our hearts through the Holy Spirit, who has been given to us."

Romans 5:3-5

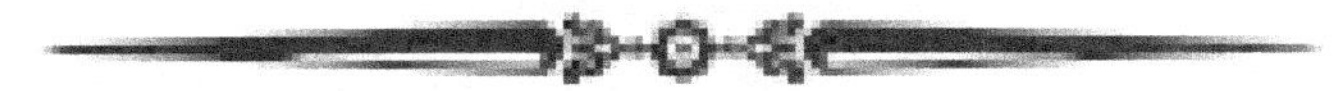

Chapter 11

STAGES OF HEALING FROM

PAIN, PROPOGATION AND PERFECTION

Healing appears like water filling a cup that spills over and reveals itself in other facets of a person's life. It has a cascading effect that will reveal limitless possibilities in your life. Healing is a push into purpose and a future. It is impossible to shift into tomorrow, strapped in the harness of yesterday's brokenness. Shout for destiny, while you reflect on your days before today's, barrenness and fruitlessness.

Can you feel it? You are on the precipice of birthing heaps of favor and blessings. It is time to think big and pursue big! Envision your vision for your future. A grand and glorious space awaits you. Don't allow people or possessions to motivate you to retreat! Lot's wife whirled into a pillow of salt, for going back. There is danger and double trouble, even possible demise in looking back. Now that the eyes of your heart have been opened, focus on being the beneficiary of healing. Healing is before you, not behind you! You must proceed to receive it!

God's vision for you, was always bigger than the vision you or people may have had for you. While you follow the direction and leading of the Holy Spirit for your life, gaze forward. Look unto the hills from whence your directives, nourishment and cure come from. Remember that your healing will not only benefit you, but generations are waiting, depending and in expectation of you.

Reestablish you!

Recreate you!

Before you were born, God laid the foundation and set the groundwork to ensure that you thrive and produce in this world, from a healthy place. What are you waiting for? You are no longer in the *waiting chamber*, not even *The Healing Chamber,* but you have transitioned to the *healed chamber!* Declare that you shall dwell and live healed, fruitful and blessed. Whatsoever you touch, and whatsoever your hands desire to do it shall transform into gold.

Create your Rehoboth place and flourish in it! God created acres of space and spans of land for you to succeed and fulfil your purpose on earth. Competition need not enter your celebration, or trespass into your thoughts. "Of David. A psalm. The earth is the LORD's, and everything in it, the world, and all who live in it; for he founded it on the seas and established it on the waters." (Psalm 24:1-

2) There is a fertile, flourishing and flush place carved out on earth for you to inhabit, possess and dominate.

Command your space!

Envision your space!

Occupy your space!

Rainy season has ended!

Barren season has been lifted!

You don't have to be downcast, revisit your abuse, the minutes of being misused, mistreated, wounded or molested. Yesterday's gone! Today is here! Use it as a springboard, to launch you, into a hope and future. Forthwith and on the double, decide that you will embrace the vision that God has crafted for you, before the foundation of the world. You overcome by the blood of the Lamb, and the word of your testimony according to Revelation 12:11. Guarantee that you will take yesterday's pain and use it to propel you into a prepared future. You were created to transcend to a place of creativity, productivity and occupancy.

All things in your life will work together, for your good. Pray unceasingly and ask God for what you desire. Verify that your desires are in alignment with His desires for your life. There are many who tried to maneuver their life without God, but ended up back at the starting line, or far-removed from it. Trust in God and He will be the best Pilot you ever encountered. God does not need a co-pilot. He is well able to navigate your life and the life of within sight of 8 billion people in His Omnipresence.

God never intended for human lives to be winding, whorled, twisted and twirled. He established a straight and narrow path for healthy, whole people to live. He purposed that people would lead unbroken, uninterrupted lives full of promises. There are countless books circulating on Motivation! There are innumerable books on Inspiration! The Bible however is inundated with De*clarations*, that you can declare over you, your family and your life daily and watch them come to pass.

The Supreme God dwells on the inside of you. God's thoughts toward you are favorable. He takes pleasure in launching you into a place of greatness and abundance. It's a spacious place! Yesterday is gone! Today is here! Tomorrow anticipates you! Liberate yourself from the mental shortcomings of yesterday and visualize yourself *breaking forth* and operating perfectly in your purpose. Lay aside every weight that beset you. Break forth from behind the brick wall and guarded space. No longer will you bury yourself and go underground, hiding from people because of shame and disgrace. "The sacrifices of God are a broken spirit; a broken and contrite heart, O God, thou will not despise." (Psalm 51:17) You have endured cycles upon cycles in your life of surviving being bruised, battered and wounded. Without delay, you are being permitted to breathe, and abide in peace.

Don't play roulette with your healing. It came at a weighted price. That helpless, weary place is prohibited from visiting your today or your future gatherings. Oh, taste and recognize that God is good. His healing endures forever. The gift of healing is to preserve, not maladminister and prodigalize. Once you have tasted of the goodness of God's restoration, remain in that place. Let the transformation that occurred, continue. Hope thou in God, to secure, and sustain you, in the restored place. The stronghold of coffee breaks, disorganization, partiality and incompleteness in your life is over. Leave and forget that familiar place, that imprisoned you persistently and incurably.

Discover people, who will travail, invest and devote time in you and akin to them. *Unhealed* people need *healed* people! They need people that will transfer a spirit of wholeness into them, to stimulate and activate their healing. People who are creating, pursuing and striving for wholeness, are the kind of people that your life deserves now.

Incline your ears unto the wise, inspired, trained and matured. Persistently seek God on your and their purpose and direction for your life. Lean unto God and acknowledge His Sovereignty in your life. When God conveys an instruction, oblige Him. Reading this book is not a fortuitous event! It is divine and orchestrated by God.

God purposed this as your healed season. Embrace this Kairos moment. This time was appointed by God! Adhere to the God breathed instruction for your life. It will prosper you! Accept here and now, that your life is shifting from the mundane to the extraordinary. This is a supernatural and not a natural moment. Embrace and hold it tightly in your arms. This present moment was created to birth you into a divine place. Your perspective shifts because your point of reference has been repositioned, toward God. Think on God! Fix your eyes upon Jesus, who is the Creator and Perfecter of your faith. He has set the prize before you, so pursue it with joy.

"Let me hear joy and gladness; let the bones you have crushed rejoice."

Psalm 51:8

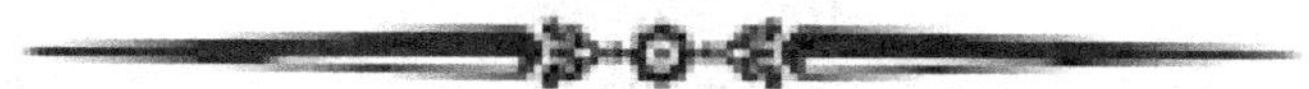

Chapter 12

AWAKENED IN HEALING

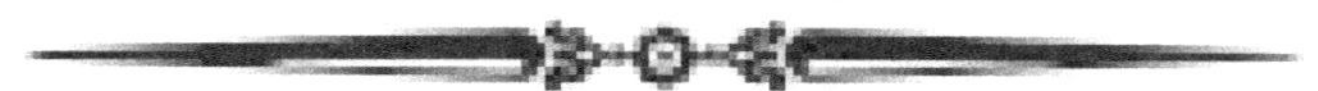

Healing is the prerequisite for wholeness! In order to heal, you must identify the source of bleeding. Whatever cut, scraped or punctured your well-being must be pinpointed. Complete wound healing requires that you interrupt and segregate from the source of your pain. Being made whole allows the wound that incapacitated you to reconstruct and reassemble completely and perfectly.

It doesn't matter anymore that your condition lingered for endless seasons. The woman with the issue of blood came to a divine place, a moment in time. She was broken-down, battered and empty. She became desperate and refused to accept the status quo, one minute longer. The noise of people and their traditions was not going to nullify her faith in Jesus. Press beyond your condition and the noise of the crowd and touch the hem of His garment. Do it NOW!

Be thou made whole!

Jesus was always cognizant of what you endured, but today He asks you the question, do you want to be healed? The invalid who had been lying at the Pool of Bethesda for thirty-eight years, in his condition answered Jesus, telling Him "Sir, I have no man to put me into the pool when the water is stirred up; but while I am coming, another steps down before me." (John 5:7) It is not unrealistic for you to expect help from others, like the sick man did. His experience some thousands of years ago, mirrors many. It epitomized mine! Yes, you may have been bypassed and overlooked. The exchange of his condition for healing occurred when Jesus showed up to help him. If the man knew how to obtain his healing before, he would not have been in that condition all those years. Immediately when he was advised by the greatest mentor of all, Jesus, to "Get up, pick up your mat, and walk.", he did. The man was healed!

Do not remain in that stupor! Emerge from the broken place.

Awaken to the rejuvenated, restored, refreshed place. Become invigorated and fired up now. God will send Jesus to come see about you; you have come face to face with the Master. Jesus commands you to Arise! Take up what was confining you and now, you carry it and walk! Get up, in this season of provision and go gather what God has prepared for you. This is your season, of perpetual healing and wholeness. Healing is yours for keeps. Don't allow anyone to make you feel like your healing is undeserved. Where were they when you lingered incomplete all those years?

I am beyond the time when the success I pursued was focused on my professional achievement, ability and acumen. This season, with much mentoring and teaching from the Holy Spirit and those that God has entrusted with my life, I have matured into what true success, really is. Time invested with God, assembled by an album collection of life experiences, have awakened me to conclude that my success lies in discovering and knowing my divine reason for being placed on this earth. Perfect dedication to pursuing destiny, coupled with being positioned in the well-defined place that God predestined, is my cup of tea now. "But seek ye first the kingdom of God, and his righteousness; and all these things shall be added unto you." (Matthew 6:33)

Awakening to your healing does not negate attacks from the enemy. The trinity of the devil will increase his pricks and prods, to seduce you into thinking you have not been healed. Additionally, he will play tricks with you and cause you to categorize one period of pain and make it applicable to your entire life. You will be revisited with whispers from the adversary with questions like: did you marry the right person? Did you choose the right career? Did you move to the right street, city or town? Could you have made better or other choices in life? Do not allow the enemy to draw you into that breathless place.

God purposed your life to be aligned and operate in homeostasis. There are moments when God will require you to be still, but you must understand what still requires. You can be still, and while still, write, plan, set goals and create a vision. God is not a God of nothingness! His plan for your life is not nothingness! In the beginning according to Genesis, the first Chapter starting at verse two, the earth was a heap of nothingness. It was formless and empty, but God's spirit hovered over the face of the waters. He spoke and commanded what was meaningless to become meaningful. What was out of equilibrium became balanced! Disorder had strict orders to shift, into divine order!

During hardship and pain the loving arms of God will comfort you as you saturate your spirit in worship. When nothingness approaches, and tries to lure you, this is the moment you must dig deep, and pull on the promises of God, which are yes and Amen for your life. "I will not leave you comfortless: I will come to you." (John 14:18) Know where to find peace and rest for your soul. In the presence of Jehovah, troubles will disappear, and your heart will be mended, in His presence.

Commit your spirit into His hands, so that He can consume the dolor. Cheer up! Let His Son shine in!

I know and understand setting forth to accomplish projects that you physically and mentally were incapacitated from pursuing, due to the temporary visibility zero-zero. Home projects, book publishing, investments, travel, all interrupted by incompleteness in life. There goes the negative cascading effect. If you do not correct one area of your life, it will infiltrate into others and cause a web of incompleteness and being unfulfilled in life. God is wise! God is specific! If He desired you to be on *Winning Boulevard* in 1990, and on *Favor Avenue* in 1993, you would have been there. He is God! Nothing can occur without Him ordaining it! God allowed the diversions, detours, deflections and digressions to process and purify you.

This book has purpose! It is on divine assignment to rescue and unleash people, from *Purposeless to Purposeful, Worthless to Worthwhile and Unfruitful to Fruitful living.*

As I sit here at 12:23a.m. typing and listening to the *"Strings of Praise Favorites"* a new day has dawned in and an old one shifted out. I declare this the *shift* of your *season*, from old to new and broken-down to healed. You have purpose Sir, Ma'am, Boy and Girl. His hand is upon you! May you experience the breath of God, blowing fresh upon you. Prophecy precedes you! The right hand of God has come to deliver and thrust you forth. Dormancy and inactivity have been apprehended. You are no longer imprisoned, by the state of your yesterday. This is a brand-new day.

God does not make mistakes. He created and formed us in His image with the innate ability to produce and pursue. Fruitfulness and favor are embedded in our DNA. Your fingerprints have been marked for success. You are of the lineage of Abraham, Isaac and Jacob. Take your fortified self and walk in your vocation, for God's glory! May every painful moment be used to display the goodness of God.

You have been healed and freed, to promote, push and unlock doors for someone else. You are a temple, not created by man's hands, but the nail scarred, hallowed hands of Jesus, the son of God. Raise your breath and praise Him! Blow your horn! Pluck the harp! Clash the cymbals, in resounding praise for everything that the Lord has brought you through.

You were carried through valleys and delivered out of wilderness experiences. The mountains and tossed sea encounters thrust you into the presence of God. None of your pain or hurt was hidden. God was only qualifying you, for your life's assignment. Had I not encountered the afflictive times in my life, the anointing that God placed upon my life, would not exist. Being tested, qualifies you to be trusted. I mastered intercession and ascended into realms and dimensions in God, which I never knew. I would not have attained it without walking through the dark seasons of my life. It pulled me directly into the fold of God. The anointing comes at a hefty price. It is extremely costly! I know all too well what being on the desert side of the mountain is. Praise God He dispatched ravens to feed me there and angelic beings to be by my side. Been there, experienced it, but I was not consumed.

Adversity, often-times is the irritant that God uses to bring people into divine position. No matter how intensely people try, they are powerless. They lack the ability to detract or withhold any blessing that God individualized to bestow upon you. Blessed be the name of the Lord! Give Reverence to God! Worship God! Renounce every opportunity to visit your yesterday. Stare boldly into the eyes of your today and focus on your glorious future. It is time to pivot in the direction of your future.

Use this weapon, this book to breakthrough and come through! The transparency of these pages is infusing its way into your spirit and agitating your purpose. I pray for the pages to jump into your spirit and change your life. "For the letter killeth, but the spirit giveth life." (2 Corinthians 3:6) Always remember the intensity with which you prayed and lamented to God, for a sign of deliverance and healing to appear. He heard you! He is speaking to you through these pages. "To the chief Musician, A Psalm of David. I waited patiently for the LORD; and He inclined unto me, and heard my cry." (Psalm 40:1)

Don't forget the hours of seeking God and pleading with Him to change the trajectory of your life. Open your mind to the possibility that God sent this opuscule, penned by His servant, to place in your hands, to jump-start your healing. I pray that this treasure resuscitates and rebirths you. I may not be your preferred Best-Selling author, but I am a chosen vessel of God, to activate this quantum leap, breakthrough moment in your life.

I declare this an outbreak, and daybreak moment in your life. Capture it! The diamond that was once muddy and being refined by fire, is beginning to shine and emerge from the ashes. Awaken, activate and vivify to your healing. Change has come, a divine shift has located you! It is crucial that you distinguish the voice of God, over human voices. A litany of celebrity, and high-profile voices may be popular, but God's voice is Supreme. Don't miss the voice of God, in this season!

As you awaken and take your healing journey, commit to sharing this renewing book of healing with as many people as possible. Gift it! Help me to share the gift of healing. The earth needs healed not broken people. Let the healing balm of Gilead permeate the earth. May it transfuse hearts, one person at a time.

When you have been revived and stirred, you understand that every wilderness and desert experience was necessary. Every positive and negative encounter was melted together, to help change the trajectory of one's life. A series of favor filled moments, have inundated my life. I thank God for those that He equipped to deposit seeds of healing in my life and filter out the clutter and refuse that was occupying precious storage space in my life.

Immerse yourself in this moment, this life transforming moment and capture every pearl that you need to jumpstart your life. Seize what God is revealing to you, through this print. Envision yourself encircled by people with successful routines who understand who they are, where they are going, and what they desire to achieve. Veto the multitude of viewpoints in your life! His instructions and directives are what you must follow.

You have experienced deceit, been bypassed and misled. Now, don't allow yourself to be placed in that position ever again. Here is a better idea, be intentional! Vow that you will never misguide or misuse another human for selfish gain. Withdraw from valuable sources and deposit where possible! Your deposit may not be intellectual, but it may be monetary or vice versa.

Learn how to honor those who invest in your growth and prosperity. "But the one who does not know and does things deserving punishment will be beaten with few blows. From everyone who has been given much, much will be demanded; and from the one who has been entrusted with much, much more will be asked." (Luke 12:48)

Your healing and wholeness have a divine purpose. Seek God on what He desires you to do with the gift of healing that He has bestowed upon you. Never forget where you surfaced from. If you covet being blessed by God, learn to return honor. The grateful heart is toward God first and then to those that invested in you. "And one of them, when he saw that he was healed, turned back, and with a loud voice glorified God, And fell down on *his* face at his feet, giving him thanks: and he was a Samaritan." (Luke 17:15-16)

"A merry heart doeth good like a medicine: but a broken spirit drieth the bones."

Proverbs 17:22

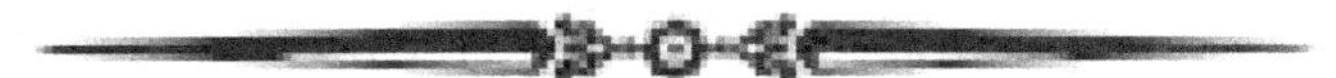

Chapter 13

THE JOY OF A HEALING SEASON

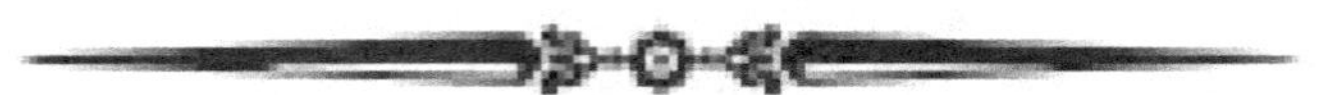

*T*he Healing Chamber was available for me! It is open for you and whomsoever will come. Healing is a wave, a supernatural force that blows, moves, and should continually flow. Joy is a fruit of healing! It has revolutionary power! Joy comes from God and healing is received from God. The Joy of the Lord is your wholeness! Joy is courageous, energizing, vitalizing and gives stability and soundness of mind, body and spirit.

In this time and season of healing, let the wave of healing increase your momentum. This writing has become an eye opener, and a valuable script, that can be applied to strengthen your life. Behold, this is your harvest season, kick-off your gathering season. Yield the parcels of blessings prepared exclusively for you. This is the season to harvest the whole shebang. It is your season to reap completeness, peace, joy and promotion. The skies are now blue, unloading in your favor. The sun is shining brighter than it ever has before. The air is refreshing and colorful, one that you can appreciate and celebrate.

The cost of the oil in your translucent box, is not measurable by humans. Flesh was not present, the days and nights you rocked in pain. The crushing and pulverizing, going through the refiner's fire was uncomfortable. Ponder with me, a sweet potato. If you taste it when it is raw, unprocessed and uncooked, it will be pleasing. When the sweet potato can go through the fire, to be processed and cooked fully, the sweetness and pleasantness magnifies. When you go through the fire and become purified, you are cleansed of impurities and your value doubles. Human preference is usually to place on the shelf the memories of unrefined times, and you should, but periodically you must open the box, as a lesson, and testimony of what you emerged from. Pulling that container from the shelf encourages one to appreciate where they are and where they emerged from. Disobedience and imprudence are contenders of healing. It's the been there, done that syndrome.

It's a new season, it's the dawn of a new day. The refreshing of being in a healed place, ought to consume you, like oxygen perfusing your airway. The wade through tumultuous waters was bloodcurdling, but you triumphed over the storm-tossed seas. Fire could not consume you, though you felt the temperature of the roaring flames, because God showed up, in the middle of the fire. Even when you could not trace Him, He held your hand invisibly through it. God knew that one day you would prevail and that you would walk in total healing.

Welcome to your spacious place. Immeasurable faith brings forth unbounded healing. God will shift the opportunities in your life, favorably. "For this light momentary affliction is preparing for us an eternal weight of glory beyond all comparison, so we do not focus on what is seen, but on what is unseen. For what is seen is temporary, but what is unseen is eternal." (1 Corinthians 4:17-18)

God has treasures stored up, just for you! Treasure hunt for your treasures. As you engage in prayer and study the Word of God, and create an intimate connection with God, He will reveal the hidden things concerning your life. Your tears are recorded in His heart, your prayers are stored in His memory. You are now redeemed! Jesus is responsible for changing your entire world.

During my moments of misfortune, my visual scope could only zoom in on what I was experiencing. It was a myopic and limited view. There were life support moments, but I still felt God's presence. The battle was real. The light of God flickered through, reminding me to recognize that change was forthcoming. He induced my womb, by showing me snippets of my reborn future. I was determined to do what was necessary to capture the beauty of the stars.

There is a scripture that my grandmother wrote on a serrated, lined piece of paper when I was preparing to leave for college in the early 1990s. The paper read, "Thy word have I hid in mine heart, that I might not sin against thee." (Psalm 119:11) Depositing God in the treasury of my heart and seeking Him while I was young, postured me. During the times that I was withdrawn, I had fragments of hope not to go off the deep end, in the recession moments of my life. Many adversities, roadblocks and bottlenecks, but I did not meet a head on collision. It was uncomfortable! The test seemed prolonged, but I procured liberal supplies of God beforehand, that was vitamin to my spirit and soul, during the unhealthy, hiccup seasons.

When you have knowledge of what awaits you, despite affliction, you will not be crushed. You will not drift from God. God's faithfulness will cause Him to incline unto you and speak into your life and situation. Serving God does not grant you immunity, it affords you resiliency. Fortify yourself in God and do not withdraw from serving God. Transcend beyond what you weathered for it was necessary. Shift your energy, gaze on the Creator and not your condition. Recognize that the people that you were hoping would help you, were merely resources. Only God has the authority and the ability to activate your life. He is the source of all things. The *torture chamber* is shut and batten down. Thank God for *the Healing Chamber* which is open. Grant God permission to order and manage your steps. Intensify your life of prayer and ascend to another level and dimension of prayer. Spend time with God, so that you may partake of the mega blessings of God. Let God teach your hands to war and your fingers to fight, so that you can break beyond the ceilings that mankind has set-up, to impede you. You have been wired to go beyond the status quo.

Everything that jeopardized your healing last season, has been captured, exposed, and defeated in this season. God's word was sent to heal your *mental, emotional, physical, financial* and *spiritual* issues. Direct your countenance toward God, you were created to prosper, not suffer. May the oxygen supply in your life, be filtered and free flowing.

Breathe in! Breathe out!

This is the season to harvest everything that went awry. This is harvest time, it is your reward season. Things are preferred and uninterrupted. The *Breaker*, your *Healer* has entered your life.

When God heals you, your countenance changes. The glory glows and it attracts. Remember anything that glitters and radiates will attract the welcomed and unwelcomed but the ultimate glory belongs to God. He must showcase His healing power and handiwork in your life, for all to witness.

The pages have turned! A new chapter has been unleashed!

The pages in your life have literally Shifted from:

- Hopeless to Hopeful
- Broken to Whole
- Poor to Rich
- Foolish to Wise
- Sick to Healed

Your imprisoned season has been commuted to your healed, whole and favored season. Barrenness has shifted to productivity. The closed doors and desert moments, where water did not seem to flow, has changed. You are now planted by rivers of water and you shall bring forth healthy and nourishing fruit in due season that will last. It's your winning season! Ascend unto the high place! The years that the worms embezzled shall be doubled unto you.

"And Jesus went about all the cities and villages, teaching in their synagogues, and preaching the gospel of the kingdom, and healing every sickness and every disease among the people."

Matthew 9:35

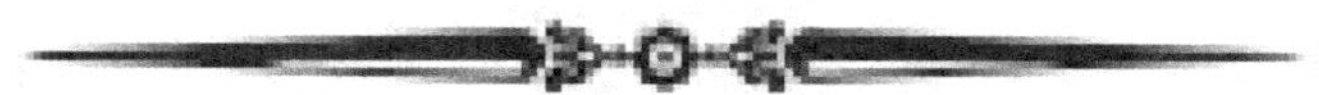

Chapter 14

EXPERT CLASSROOM OF HEALING

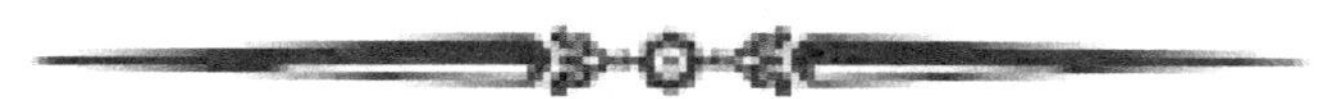

Life is a classroom with many teaching moments. It is a journey that requires emotional, mental and spiritual strength. Emotional hurt carries so many emotions, including displeasure, frustration, bafflement and feelings of being unfulfilled. There are many battles that humans face on their life sojourn such as anxiety, unforgiveness, depression, oppression, grief, loss, remorse, abuse, misuse and mistreatment. Whatever kind of struggle life presents you, there is light at the end of the tunnel.

In the classroom of life, there is one major lesson that pain teaches you, and that is patience. The time that you spent in the process worketh patience on the inside of you. "Knowing this, that the trying of your faith worketh patience." (James 1:3)

Rejoice in your trials because perseverance matures and completes you. Mastering patience qualifies you for healing and the promises of God.

The classroom of life is ever filled with enlightenment and lessons that you are meant to learn. You must be willing to submit to the teacher, invest the time and work, so that you may obtain the lessons needed to graduate. Isn't it amazing that you could occupy a seat in a classroom filled with diverse students with various issues and vicissitudes of life! In the natural classroom of life, it is possible to be overlooked especially when you are not performing optimally.

The *Rabbi* of all *Rabbi's* knows your name. You can never go unrecognized to Him. Somewhere in the classroom of life, you remembered the still small voice, that whispered to you that *"I know your name."* Your gift was being fortified and magnified. At the appointed time, your name will be called. The earth has need of you!

It is now your set time to shift from faith to faith and go from glory to glory. God was with you in the valley and awaits you on the mountaintop. What was inside of you was always worthy, that was why the enemy fought you tooth and nail, because he knew the value of what you carried. What was meant to bruise you didn't consume you, rather it fortified you, so as to launch you into the most profitable and prosperous season of your life. God turned it! Stronger and wiser that's you!

Surge ahead into your upraised and uplifted season. You could not access your spacious place prematurely. It was the Lord's doing, that He held you in the *waiting chamber* until it was the set time for you to give birth to your promise.

Every human has needs ranging from basic such as food and shelter to complex which include a sense of personal value and accomplishment. Human love from friends and people are not to be downplayed. When a human lacks self-fulfillment and falls short of their full potential, that can leave a person unfulfilled, sad and ungratified about any and all things. However, God desires people to be purpose and pursuit driven. This is the order of healing. Every aspect of human needs must be realized.

Unaccomplished people are fragmented people!

Yesterday was the pushups, squats and drill warm-ups for this season. The conditioning was imperative to boost you to matriculate to the next level. There must be an awakening in your soul, from the moments of investigation and training, to manifestation of the promises of God. Your elected and set apart season was preceded by your gestation and anticipation season. When you enter your favored and approved season, do not revert to the memories, of the drill season. Let the past go! Devote your thoughts and creativity to the present and future season. God is a present help in the time of trouble. He has promised to heal. It is crucial to remain motivated and not clouded by the memory of aforetime.

Know when to invest in self! One day I stepped out on faith and pursued my *Master of Arts Degree in Theology*. At a God ordained time, I sacrificed to attend an *Impartation* gathering, which RESET my entire life. The divine impartation shifted me mentally, spiritually, emotionally and mentally. That was a regenerating moment for me. My breathing pattern began to normalize! My heart rate became regular once again. Vigor returned to my step! I had not felt that refreshed in a long time. I had to cross the water for that moment to occur. Miracles are connected to water. The healing power of God was injected into me and there was a rebirth on the inside of me. It is graduation season! Your cap and gown have been prepared for you! You dared to walk into *The Healing Chamber* and touch the hem of His garment, now you have been made whole.

A natural classroom, infused with a supernatural lesson, changed my life. Rays of light radiated through and happiness began to fill my spirit once again. Vision and passion reclaimed me, afresh. The concept of a mentor is misunderstood! It is a gift to every human! Pray and seek God on who your mentor is. Locate them, and your life will change forever!

Mentorship is vitality! A mentor presents you a picture of what your future will look like. Everyone should have a voice in their life that they find trustworthy. The Holy Spirit is the ultimate teacher, however God gifted one or more humans with what you need to go to the next level in life. A mentor helps you to navigate life, using their wisdom, training and experience. Pose questions! Listen and follow their instructions.

You were created on purpose, for purpose. People are waiting on your artistry, genius and formulas. Operate in your exclusivity, and let God release you into peculiar places, where people have been waiting on you. Preserve and protect your healing. Sashay in your wholeness!

Son, daughter walk across the stage and receive your diploma. You have been awarded certificate Summa Cum Laude in *"Unending Lessons in Life Instructed by God."* Receive it, with your head held high! You earned it lawfully! Your stripes and battle scars are proof!

"Then He said to her, "Daughter, your faith has healed you.
Go in peace."

Luke 8:48

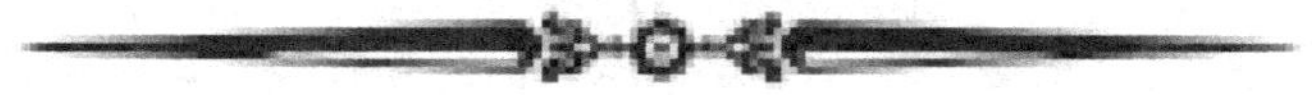

Chapter 15

PRESERVE AND PERPETUATE YOUR HEALING

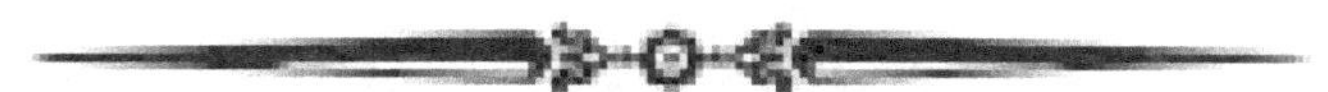

What you earned at a price should be nurtured and preserved. Keep, manage, protect and nurture your healing. Anything that interferes with your ability to breathe, and live in a healed space, must be resisted, repelled and rejected. Remember when you were broken, your breathing pattern, and ability to fully inhale and exhale were compromised. A challenged breath was an opponent to your power, compass and range of motion. Life has been reset mentally, emotionally, physically and spiritually. You are now in a revised, rise and shine space. Establish and settle there! Hold tightly your healing and focus on your restored, revivified and harmonized season.

Saunter in power!

Guard your space and protect your peace. Be careful to discern who desires to abide in your life. Seek God on their purpose and posture in your life. Be very intentional about maintaining your wholeness. Be aware that while you strive to preserve your healing, adversity will present itself.

This time, you will have the memory cells of your past season and the antibodies to repel the sight and smell of any antigen that is attempting to inflame and infect your life, once again. Your *waiting chamber* was your *preparation chamber* for God's *Healing Chamber*. I pray that you will be spirit lead, and not emotionally moved.

Take your life experiences and use it as a classroom for those that you connect with. Your experiences were not only for you, but for those you are purposed to guide, nourish and support. Exist creatively and full of vigor. Live gratefully and steadfastly, immovable, but abounding in God.

Nourish your healing!

Modus to maintain your Healing

- Study the Word of God
- Believe His promises for your life
- Increase your faith
- Trust God
- Be truthful with you
- Remain in intimate relationship with God

Maintain an environment in your life, surrounded by other like-minded people. Preserve your space and secure your surroundings. Say no, to anything and anyone that endangers your peace, healthy and sound mind. Healing has a formula, keep the secrets! Stay connected to God. Be directed by the Holy Spirit. Jesus heals! Jesus delivers! Jesus makes whole! I pray that my transparency births your healing. *The Healing Chamber* is where you encounter God.

I pray that this was a well-timed writing peering into seasons of my life of holding pattern and waiting path, reflecting into yours and the imperfection, setbacks and miscarriages. It was a glimpse into my mountain and valley experiences and how they have crafted me, into a complete vessel that was now qualified to tell my story and be a source of healing, breakthrough and strength for you. My unwished-for rest was purposeful in preparing me to *enrich, equip, empower, mentor, birth* and *activate* souls. It is my prayer that this spirit guided penning has sparked the process of healing toward wholeness in your life.

Life is comprised of undulation and rotations, which are undesired and unmelodious, but ultimately it shall reveal purpose. This book was not only a weapon to activate healing in broken humans, but it was my journey, as the first partaker of a bona fide transformation.

The greatest declarations for your life can be found in the Word of God!

The Word of God is:

- Proven
- Effective
- Trustworthy
- Unimpeachable

Open it!

Declare it!

Walk in your total Healing!

"If my people, which are called by my name, shall humble themselves, and pray, and seek my face, and turn from their wicked ways; then will I hear from heaven, and will forgive their sin, and will heal their land."

2 Chronicles 7:14

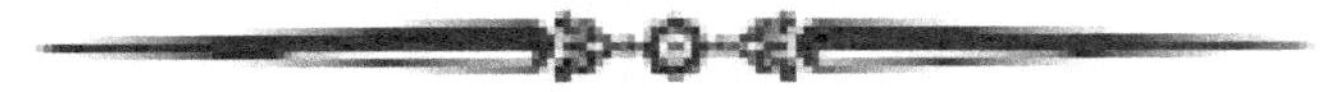

Chapter 16

PRAY YOUR WAY TO HEALING

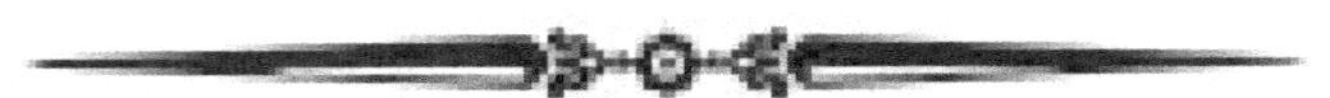

You possess the ability to pray your way into healing. You must know how to posture yourself in prayer so that perpetual healing can flow in every area of your life. Prayer is practical, but it is powerful and transformative.

We all have areas of our lives that need healing such as emotional, physical, financial, marital and even spiritual healing. There are countless people traversing the earth, that have endured a kind of hurt that is unclassified and indescribable. It is proliferating the earth, and I tag it as *"institution hurt."* This is volumes of books unto itself. Many people are broken and unable to understand that their bitterness lies in what they interpret or experienced being part of an institution. They were cut deeper than they can comprehend or verbalize. These souls need healing and restoration.

If we occupy space on this earth, we must position ourselves in prayer so that we can walk in healing. There are limitless amounts of people walking the earth, who need to pray morning, night and noon for healing.

You need to Posture in earnest Prayer:

1. If you may have been in a barren, unproductive state for years upon years, and you have no idea how to break the cycle.

2. If you may have dismissed the precepts and principles that God outlined, hence you ended up far from what He promised for you and your life.

3. When you identify that earthly riches cannot seem to find and stay in your hands.

4. When everyone around you appears to be prospering, but you are not experiencing any signs of prosperity in your life.

5. When sickness and disease seem to constantly plague you.

6. When no dots seem to be able to connect in your life and there is lack of success.

7. When cyclical issues are evident in your life.

8. When you sense that diabolic spirits are attacking you in multiple areas of your life.

9. If you have been experiencing season after season of despair.

Simply because you are accustomed to walking in barrenness and disorder for a long time, does not mean that your healing will not be realized. When you are healed, your entire life will begin to shift. You must pursue your healing in order to walk in a purpose filled life. Intercede and supplicate for your complete healing.

This world was crafted by God's hands but there is an influence, a power that operates in opposition to God, on assignment to pull you away from your destiny. God never intended you to fight and wrestle to live in peace, be well, succeed and win. This takes many people by surprise when they face conflict, shortcomings, affliction and forces that fight against their purpose.

Prayer will posture you for God to rearrange, rebirth and reset your life. Seek out what God desires you to do, where He wants you to be, what He wants you speaking so that He has free range to move. Do the preliminary work that is required for you to be healed. No matter how worthless and woeful your story may have been, your situation can change. For healing and wholeness to touch your life, you must be willing to give up the issues that have attached itself to your condition.

Are you ready?

God is not like man!

He cannot and will not lie!

Your life can be a story for mankind to see as God can literally use you to defy human odds and put you on display for all to see the healing and transformative power of God in your life. God will raise you up to dimensions far above what you suffered and endured. Be willing to disassociate yourself from fetters of misfortune that have plagued your life.

When you recognize that you need healing and that healing is available to you, then you can walk in it. You can only have healing, if you understand that you need it. Pray and seek God for your healing. Identify your unfertile and unfortunate state. It does not matter if you were born into your condition or whether you once partook in success and lost it, you can realize it once again. Refuse to allow ducks to keep you trapped in a place, where your energy, creativity and zeal to succeed is choked. Identify with the eagle that is hiding deep on the inside of you and begin to rise, stretch and lengthen. Pray unceasingly for your healing. Get ready for your quantum leap!

Sin is common for the condition that people find themselves in. It is many times the fault of the person, or someone connected to them from a generational standpoint that they are not aware of that caused them to be in the state that they are in.

Clear the way for God to restore unto you what the locust, palmer, caterpillar and every other worm embezzled from you. Humble yourself, pray, repent and seek the face of God so that you can experience the restoration power of God in your life. A broken and contrite heart, God will not despise.

When your hands are clean and your heart is pure, when you pray to God, He will hear you and He will answer you. The purity of your heart will favor healing in every breadth of your life. It is His hope, His prayer that all is well in your life and that you are healthy in body as you are strong in spirit. If you are going to cry out to God and call forth to Him to extend his healing touch in your life, ensure that you are perfect, upright and virtuous. This is how you will excite Him to respond to your prayer.

Live right, so that God can respond right!

Prayer will unleash the healing power of God in your life. Prayer will connect you with God and provide uninterrupted connection between you and Rapha. Believe when you pray, and you shall receive! Be strategic and specific with your requests to God. Say yes to His will and to His way and His answer will be yes to you! May the healing virtue of God be expedited in your life.

Only God can take your yesterday and remodel it, thrusting you into the world as a restored, upgraded vessel, to display to the earth. In the words of *Women Breaking Forth*, may you *Break Forth* with power and demonstration of the *Healed* virtue of God.

To everything there is a season, and a time to every purpose under the heaven: A time to be born, and a time to die; a time to plant, and a time to pluck up that which is planted; A time to kill, and a time to <u>HEAL</u>; a time to break down, and a time to build up; A time to weep, and a time to laugh; a time to mourn, and a time to dance; A time to cast away stones, and a time to gather stones together; a time to embrace, and a time to refrain from embracing; A time to get, and a time to lose; a time to keep, and a time to cast away; A time to rend, and a time to sew; a time to keep silence, and a time to speak; A time to love, and a time to hate; a time of war, and a time of peace.

Ecclesiastes 3:1-8

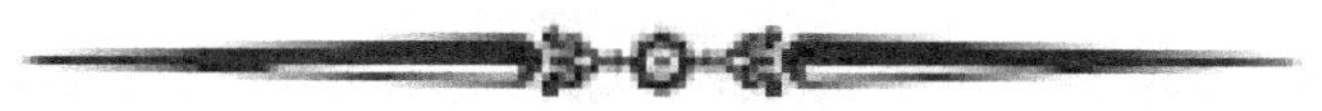

"Life is a classroom! God is the Master Teacher! Periodically, you will be afforded time to prepare for a test, other times there will be an impromptu test. The test can be swift, or prolonged, based on your response. Only the teacher can determine, whether you have been preparing, or whether you require additional preparation, to graduate to the next level!"

Tamonya Sands, M.D.

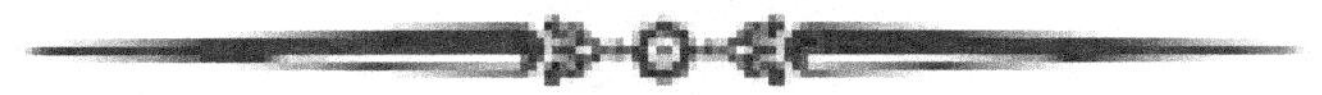

About the Author

Dr. Tamonya Sands is a wife, mother, author, speaker, physician and coach who was born and raised in the Bahamas. She has ministered and spoken locally and internationally. She has a Medical Degree from St. Matthews University School of Medicine, Grand Cayman, British West Indies since 2005. She also holds a Master of Arts in Theology from New Covenant University located in St. Augustine, Florida. She is the founder of Women Breaking Forth Global Ministries which has an Academy. Dr. Sands has served as a Professor at several colleges and held the position of Medical Chair. Dr. Sands resides in the Miami, Florida with her husband Thomas, and their princess Ashera.

9 798552 406647